AF430919

Community Pharmacy:
Basic Principles and Concepts

Community Pharmacy:
Basic Principles and Concepts

Kamal Dua

Lecturer, Department of Pharmaceutical Technology
School of Pharmacy and Allied Health Sciences,
International Medical University,
Kuala Lumpur-57000, Malaysia

Kavita Pabreja

Lecturer, Department of Life Sciences
School of Pharmacy and Allied Health Sciences,
International Medical University,
Kuala Lumpur-57000,Malaysia

Vijay Kumar Sharma

Asst. Professor, Dept. of Pharmaceutical Chemistry
D.J. College of Pharmacy, Modinagar, U.P.-201204, India

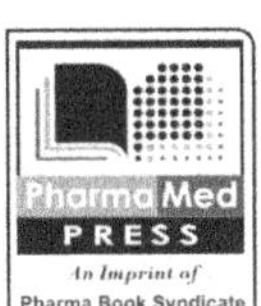

PharmaMed Press

An imprint of Pharma Book Syndicate

A unit of BSP Books Pvt. Ltd.

4-4-309/316, Giriraj Lane,
Sultan Bazar, Hyderabad - 500 095.

Published by

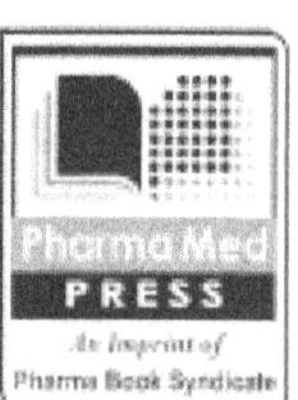

PharmaMed Press

An imprint of Pharma Book Syndicate

A unit of BSP Books Pvt. Ltd.

4-4-309/316, Giriraj Lane, Sultan Bazar, Hyderabad - 500 095.

Phone: 040-23445600, 23445688; Fax: 91+40-23445611

E-mail: info@pharmamedpress.com

ISBN: 978-93-5433-09-2 (HB)

With Eternal Gratitude
to
Almighty
and
My Family

Preface

The *"Community Pharmacy: Basic Principles & Concepts"* may suggest new ideas and thoughts to a pharmacist to help him/her in redefining the role of community pharmacist in the changing global scenario. The manuscript essentially encompasses various topics of interest in Community Pharmacy including detailed discussion on various recent topics of significance like pharmacoepidemology, pharmacoeconomics, OTC medications, health screening services; rational drug therapy which are proving potential and thrust areas as far as Community Pharmacy is concerned.

This book has been written strictly according to the curriculum of B.Pharm students of U.P. Technical University; Lucknow. It also suits to and caters the needs of medico legal professionals and may serve as text book of pharmacy students of various universities as the selected topic forms an important part of the curricula of their courses. This book provides an explicit and elaborated introduction to the fundamental principles of community pharmacy and hence helps in understanding the concepts involved in a better and effective way.

Particular emphasis has been laid down in explaining the terms and topics in simple language and in an easily understandable fashion so that students may be able to gain maximum knowledge of the subject in less time. The authors are hopeful that this book may provide awareness and create enthusiasm on the subject and useful for in-house training of the community pharmacist.

To my numerous students, whom I cannot possibly name individually, I express my sincere thanks for their class interactions which have been the guiding spirit in selection of the subject matter and its logical arrangement. We are also very much pleased in extending our sincere thanks to all who supported us and contributed in one way or the other in making our dreams true in the form of the present book. The authors are of the opinion that the suggestions, comments and criticisms at the end of the readers will help in improving the further editions of the text and such precious feed back from readers shall be highly appreciated.

- Authors

Contents

UNIT 1
INTRODUCTION AND COMMUNITY PHARMACY MANAGEMENT

Unit 2

Prescription and Inventory Control

UNIT 3

COMMUNICATION SKILLS, PHARMACEUTICAL CARE, PATIENT COUNSELING AND COMPLIANCE

UNIT 4

OTC MEDICATIONS AND HEALTH SCREENING SERVICES

Unit 5

Health Education

UNIT 6

PHARMACOECONOMICS AND PHARMACOEPIDEMIOLOGY

UNIT 7

RATIONAL DRUG THERAPY

INTRODUCTION AND COMMUNITY PHARMACY MANAGEMENT

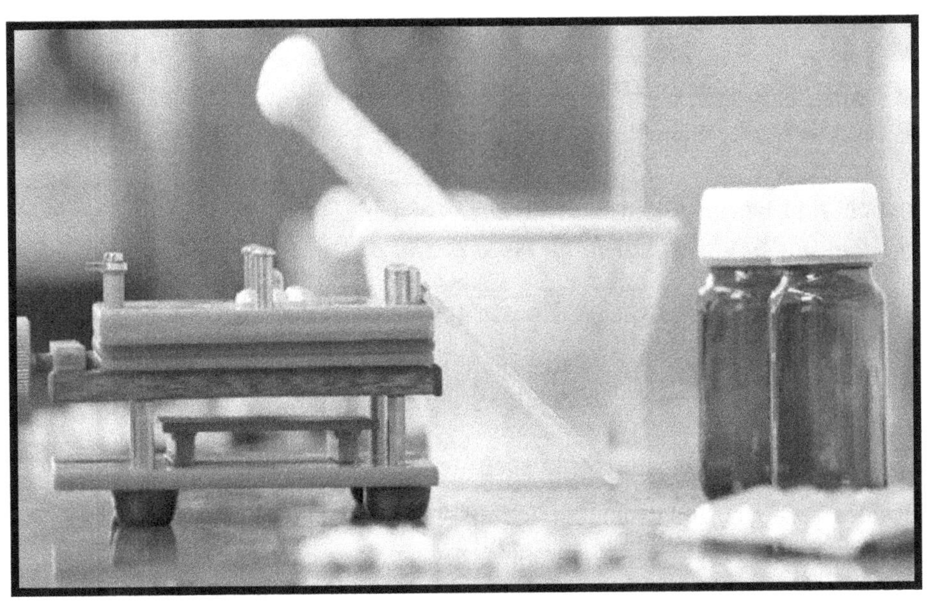

1.1   COMMUNITY PHARMACY

1.1.1 Definition

The main responsibilities of a community pharmacy include *compounding, counseling,* and dispensing of drugs to the patients with care, accuracy, and legality along with the proper procurement, storage, dispensing and documentation of medicines. The community pharmacist must be a qualified and pertinent with sound education, skills and competence to deliver the professional service to the community.

A community pharmacist should

(i)   have a sound background of pharmaceutical care, pharmacotherapy, and health promotion.

(ii)   have good communication skills with patients and other healthcare providers.

(iii)   maintain a high degree of standard in products, services, and communication.

(iv)   record and maintain his documents in order.

"In short community pharmacy is the drug use, control and effective application of knowledge of ethics, that assures optimal drug safety in the distribution and use of medicines and hence, it ensures maximum well-being of patients while they are on drug therapy."

Community Pharmacy is defined broadly to include all those establishment that are privately owned and whose function, in varying degrees is to serve societies needs for both drug product and pharmaceutical service. It is the branch of pharmacy that deals with different aspects of *patient care, dispensing of drugs and advising patient on the safe and rational drug use.*

1.1.2 Scope of Community Pharmacy

Community Pharmacy has a large number of scopes or approaches, which are related to patient counseling and patient drug control.

1.1.2.1 Drug information about their action

Besides proper understanding of the biological and physical science, community pharmacy also provides grasp on chemistry, pharmacology, toxicology, routes of administration, stability and other information regarding drugs.

The community pharmacy is an excellent institute and an educational laboratory for physician and pharmacist carrying out an obligation to provide necessary and fully authoritative information on drug. Community pharmacy acquires the knowledge by personal and individual contacts with the physician but also from the pharmacy and therapeutic committee. Community pharmacy also ensures the pharmaceutical quality of drugs and dispensing of drugs and also responsible in selection of a suitable product in the market.

1.1.2.2 Drug utilization

Community pharmacy helps to develop charging policies for pharmaceutical services. It should also be able to implement an adequate system for stock and inventory control. Community pharmacy also decides the proper regimen of drug to the patient. It also gives the knowledge to how to administer the drug to the patient.

Stock control reports on prescription and controlled drugs dispensed, drug purchases, inspection and improvement in operation and such other aspect which demand attention.

1.1.2.3 Drug distribution

Considerable quantities of drugs are localized physically outside the pharmacy. It is necessary to have control for internal distribution of drugs for patients. The patients who are hospitalized may require intensive drug therapy, controlled procedures which will allow rapid rechecks of drug source and quality. The potentialities of automated dispensing at the wards level bring further emphasis to establishment of correct controls for drug distribution in this situation.

1.1.2.4 Drug selection

In the field of community pharmacy the 'rational drug therapy' plays a important role for the selection of drugs which will be given to the patients to encounter the disease. It is defined as the use of an appropriate, efficacious, safe and cost-effective drug given for the right indication, in the right dose and at right interval of time and for the right duration of time (Dosage regimen).

It involves various type of activities like-

    (a) Adoption of essential drugs concept

    (b) Training of health professionals (counseling of health in Rational Drug Therapy/ Rational Drug Use)

    (c) Maintenance of data based on clinical guidelines

(d) Consumer education and regulatory strategies if the Rational Drug Use (RDU) is not proper it leads to illness, adverse drug reactions (ADRs), increase cost of medication and treatment to the patient.

It is also known as "Essential Drug Concept" (EDC).

1.1.2.5 Patient counseling and evaluating

Dialogues between patients and physicians regarding the indication, proper use and potential adverse effects of non-prescription drugs (NPDs) should be different as compared, when if the physician has written the prescription. In the era, the cost considerations are greater than ever, NPDs should be considered and referred when appropriate, as alternatives to prescription drugs.

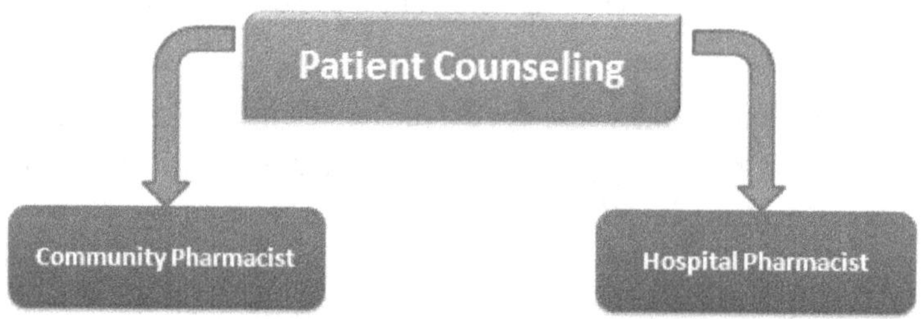

Fig. 1.1 Pharmacists involved in patient counseling

1.1.3 Role and Responsibilities of Pharmacist

(I) Central Pharmacists Responsibilities

A. *Dispensing area*

1. Ensures that established policies and procedures are followed.
2. Checks for the accuracy of doses prepared
   (a) Intravenous admixtures
   (b) Unit dose
3. Provides for proper drug control
   (a) Ensures that drugs are stored and dispensed properly (eg. Investigational drugs)
   (b) Ensure that all state and federal drug laws are followed
4. Ensure that good techniques are used in compounding intravenous admixtures and extemporaneous preparations

5. Provides for proper record keeping and billing

    (a) Patient-medication records

    (b) Extemporaneous compounding records

    (c) Intravenous admixture records billing

    (d) Investigational-drug records

    (e) Reports (eg. Monthly workload report)

6. Maintains professional competence, particularly in knowledge of drug stability and incompatibilities.

7. Ensures that new personnel are trained properly in the policies and procedures of the dispensing area.

8. Co-ordinates the activities of the area with the available staff to make the best possible use of personnel and resources.

9. Keeps the dispensing area neat and orderly.

10. Communicates with all pharmacy staff regarding new development in the area and assists in employee evaluations.

11. Provides drug information as necessary to the pharmacy, medical and nursing staffs.

12. Co-ordinates the overall pharmaceutical needs of the patients care areas with the dispensing area (eg. Delivery schedules).

B. *Patient-care area*

1. Supervision of drug administration.

    (a) Reviews and interprets each unit doses and intravenous (IV) admixture medication order to ensure that it is entered accurately into the unit-dose or IV- admixture system.

    (b) Reviews each patients drug administration form periodically to ensure that all doses are being administered and charted correctly.

2. Reviews all doses missed, reschedule the doses as necessary and signs all drugs not given notices.

3. Ensures that new drug administration forms are transcribed accurately for continuity of drug therapy and that drug charges are assessed correctly.

    (a) Confirms periodically that administered doses are noted correctly on the patient chart.

   (b) Ensures that records for administered narcotics are kept correctly and that the physician is informed of all automatics stop orders.

   (c) Ensures that proper drug administration techniques are used.

   (d) Acts as liaison between the pharmacist, the nursing and medical staffs.

   (e) Communicates with nurses and physicians concerning medication administration problems.

   (f) Periodically inspects the medication area on the nursing units to ensure that adequate levels of floor stocks drugs and supply are maintained.

   (g) Ensure that order supportive services performed from the dispensing area as required.

   (h) Ensure that the other supportive services performed by the department of pharmacy are carried out correctly.

   (i) Co-ordinate all pharmacy services on the nursing unit level.

   (j) Ensure that the medication area is neat and orderly.

   (k) Ensure that proper security is maintained in the medication area to prevent pilferage.

C. *Direct patient care*

Identifies drug brought into the hospital by patients.

Obtain patient medication histories and communicates all pertinent information to the physician.

1. Assists in drug-product and entity selection.

2. Assists the physician in selecting dosage regimens and schedules and then assigns drug administration times for these schedules (pharmacokinetic service).

3. Monitors patient s' total drug therapy for-

   (a) Effectiveness/ ineffectiveness

   (b) Side-effects

   (c) Toxicities

   (d) Allergic drug reactions

   (e) Drug interaction

   (f) Appropriate therapeutic outcomes

4. Counsels patients on

   (a) medication to be self administered in the hospital

   (b) Discharge medications

5. Participates in cardiopulmonary emergencies by

   (a) Procuring and preparing the drug required.

   (b) Charting all medications given.

   (c) Performing cardiopulmonary resuscitation, if necessary.

D. *General responsibilities*

1. Provides education to

   (a) Pharmacists, pharmacy externs, clerks, students, residents and other students.

   (b) Nurses and nursing students.

   (c) Physicians and medical students.

2. Provides drug information to physicians, nurses and other health-care personnel.

(II) Ambulatory Pharmacists Responsibilities

A. *Dispensing area*

1. Ensure that established policies and procedures are followed

2. Checks for the accuracy in the work of supportive personnel

3. Ensure that proper techniques are used in extemporaneous compounding

4. Maintenance of adequate record keeping and billing

   (a) Patient medication records

   (b) Investigational drug records

   (c) Outpatients billing

   (d) Reports

   (e) Prescription files

5. Maintains professional competence

6. Ensure that new personnel are trained properly in the policies and procedures of the ambulatory pharmacy.

7. Co-ordinate the activities of the area with available staff to make the best use of personnel and resources.

8. Keeps the ambulatory pharmacy area neat and orderly at all times.

B. *Patient care area*

1. Inspects the medication areas in the nursing unit periodically to ensure an adequate supply of stock drugs and their proper storage.

2. Identifies the drugs brought into the clinic by patients.

3. Obtains patients medication histories and communicates pertinent information to the physician.

4. Assists in drug-product entity selection.

5. Assists the physician in selecting dosage regimens and schedules.

6. Monitors the patients total drug therapy for:
   (a) Effectiveness
   (b) Side-effects
   (c) Toxicities
   (d) Allergic drug reactions
   (e) Drug interactions
   (f) Appropriate patient outcomes

7. Counsels patients on the proper use of their medications.

8. Prepare medications for intravenous administration.

9. Provides medication and/or supply for patient home care.

C. *General responsibilities*

1. Provides drug information necessary to pharmacy, medicals and nursing staffs.

2. Co-ordinates overall pharmaceutical needs of the ambulatory service area.

3. Provides adequate drug controls
   (a) Ensures that the drugs are handled properly (eg. Investigational-drug storage).
   (b) Ensures that all state and federal laws are followed

4. Maintains professional competence in area.

5. Participates in cardiopulmonary emergencies by
   (a) Procuring and preparing the drug required.
   (b) Charting all medications given.
   (c) Performing cardiopulmonary resuscitation, if necessary.

6. Provides in-service education to

   (a) Pharmacists, pharmacy externs, clerks, students, residents and other students.

   (b) Nurses and nursing students.

   (c) Physicians and medical students.

In a small hospital with only one pharmacist it is a challenge to be knowledgeable in all the activities of the hospital pharmacy. In large hospital with a number of pharmacists who specialize in certain areas of practice, each may become expert in one or more fields.

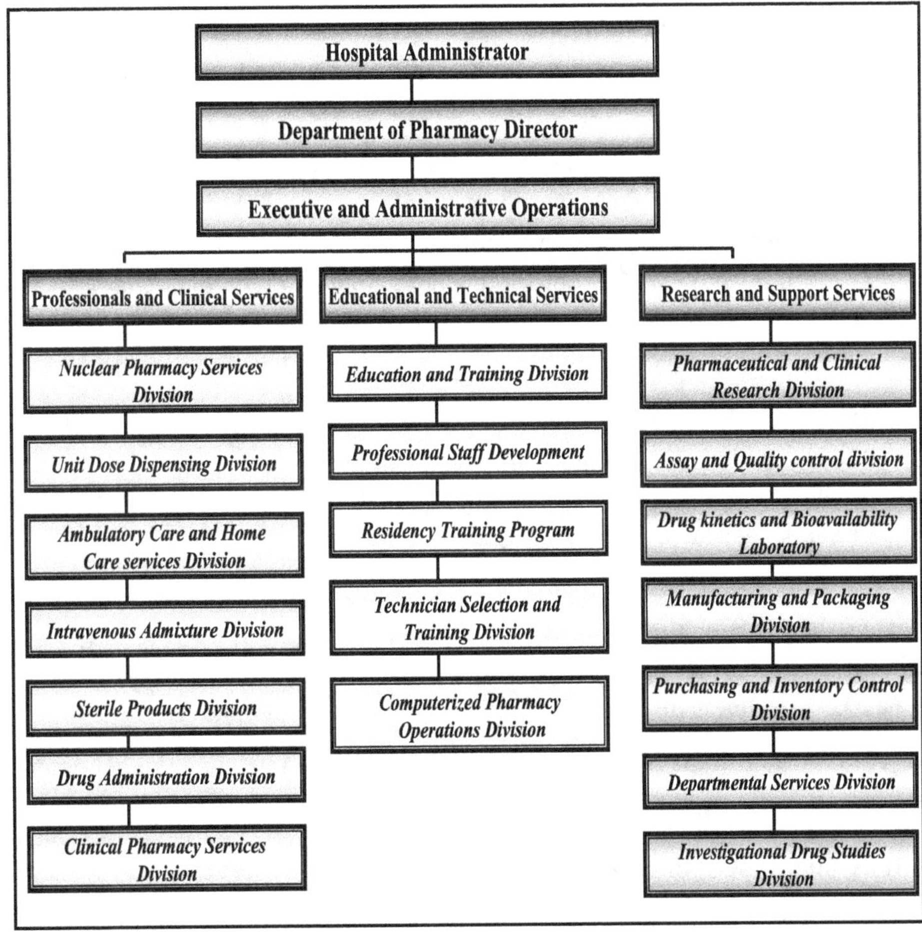

Fig. 1.2 Typical Organizational Structure of a Pharmacy Department

1.1.4 Code of Pharmaceutical Ethics

As adopted by Pharmacy Council of India under chapter-I: General Introduction, The profession of pharmacy is noble in its ideals and pious in its character. Apart from being a career for earning livelihood it has inherent in it the attitude of service and sacrifice in the interests of the suffering humanity. In handling, selling, distributing, compounding and dispensing medical substances including poisons and potent drugs a pharmacist is, in collaboration with medical men and others, charged with the onerous responsibility of safeguarding the health of people, as such he has to uphold the interests of his patrons above all things. The lofty ideals set up by Charaka, the ancient Philosopher Physician and Pharmacist in his erunciation : "Even if your own life be in danger you should not betray or neglect the interests of your patients" should be fondly cherished by all Pharmacist.

Government restricts the practice of Pharmacy to those who qualify under regulatory requirements and grant them privileges necessarily denied to others. In return Government expects the Pharmacist to recognise his responsibilities and to fulfill his professional obligations honorably and with due regard for the well being of Society.

Standards of professional conduct for pharmacy are necessary in the public interest to ensure an efficient pharmaceutical service. Every pharmacist should not only be willing to play his part in giving such a service but should also avoid any act or omission which would prejudice the giving of the services or impair confidence in any respect for pharmacists as a body.

The nature of pharmaceutical practice is such that its demands may be beyond the capacity of the individual to carry out or to carry out as quickly or as efficiently as the needs of the public require. There should, therefore at all times, be a readiness to assist colleagues with information or advice.

A Pharmacist must, above all be a good citizen and must uphold and defend the laws of the state and the Nation.

1.1.4.1 Pharmacist in relation to his job

1.1.4.1.1 *Scope of pharmaceutical service:* When premises are registered under statutory requirements and opened as a pharmacy, reasonably comprehensive pharmaceutical services should be provided. This involves the supply of commonly required medicines of this nature without undue delay. It also involves willingness to furnish emergency supplies at all times.

1.1.4.1.2 *Conduct of the pharmacy*: It should be clear to the public that practices of Pharmacy are carried out in the establishment. Signs, notices, description, which do not or imply pharmaceutical qualifications, should be limited to those of which the use is restricted by law. A notice stating that dispensing under employees by government is carried out may be exhibited at the premises. In every pharmacy, there should be a pharmacist in personal control of pharmacy that will be regarded as primarily responsible for the observance of proper standards of conduct in connection with it.

1.1.4.1.3 *Handling of prescriptions:* A prescription is presented for dispensing; it should be received by a pharmacist without any discussion or comment over it, regarding the merits and demerits of its therapeutic efficacy. In case of any error in it, due to any omission, incompatibility or over dosage, the prescription should be referred back to the presciber.

1.1.4.1.4 *Fair trade practice:* No attempt should be made to capture the business of a contemporary by cut throat competitions that are by offering any sort of prizes or gift. Label trade marks and other signs and symbols of contemporaries should not be imitated or copied.

1.1.4.1.5 *Purchase of drug:* Drug should be purchased from genuine and reputable source and a pharmacist should always be on if guard not to aid or abet, directly or indirectly.

1.1.4.1.6 *Hawking of drug:* Hawking of drugs and medicinals should not be encouraged, not should any attempt be made to solicit orders for such substances from door to door.

1.1.4.1.7 *Advertising and display*

(a) Any wording design or illustration reflecting unfavorably on pharmacist collectively or upon any group of individual.

(b) Misleading or exaggerated statements or claims.

(c) A guarantee of therapeutic efficacy.

(d) An appeal to fear.

(e) A prize competition or similar scheme.

(f) For correction or approval of the change suggested.

1.1.4.1.8 *Handling of drug:* All possible care should be taken to dispense a prescription correctly by weighing and measuring all ingredients. Incorrect proportion by the help of scales and measures, visual estimation must be avoided. A pharmacist should always use drugs and medicinal preparations of standard quality. He should never fill his prescription with spurious sub-standard and unethical preparation.

1.1.4.1.9 *Apprentice pharmacist:* While incharge of a dispensary, drug store or hospital pharmacy where apprentice pharmacist are admitted for practical training. A pharmacist should see that the trainees are given full facilities for their work, so that on the completion of their training they have acquired sufficient technique and skill to neck themselves dependable pharmacist.

1.1.4.2 Pharmacist in relation to his trade

1.1.4.2.1 *Price structure***:** Price charged from customers should be fair and in keeping with the quality and quantity of commodity supplied and the labor and skill required in making it ready for use.

1.1.4.3 Pharmacist in relation to medical profession

1.1.4.3.1 *Limitation of professional activity:* Whereas it is expected that practitioners in general would not take to practice of pharmacy by owing drug stores as this ultimately leads to coded prescriptions and monopolistic, detrimental to the pharmaceutical profession and also to the interest of patients; it should be made a general rule that pharmacist under no circumstances, take to medical practices that is diagnosing diseases and prescribing remedies, therefore even if requested patrons do so.

No pharmacist should recommend particular medical practitioner unless specifically ask to do so.

1.1.4.3.2 *Clandestine arrangements:* No pharmacist should enter into any secret arrangements or conduct with the physician, to offer him any commission or any advantage by recommending his dispensary or drug store himself to the patients.

1.1.4.3.3 *Liaison with public:* Being a liaison between medical profession and people, a pharmacist should always keep himself abreast with the modern developments in pharmacy and other periodicals.

1.1.4.4 Pharmacist in relation to his profession

It is not sufficient for a pharmacist to be law abiding and to deter from doing things derogatory to the society and his profession, but it should be his duty to make others also fulfill the provisions of the pharmaceutical and other law regulations.

1.1.4.4.1 *Law-abiding citizen:* A pharmacist is a unit whole and his life cannot be divided into compartments. A pharmacist, engaged in profession has to be an enlightened citizen endowed with a fair knowledge of the law of the land and he should be particularly conversant with the enactments pertaining to food, drug, pharmacy, health, sanitation and the like and endeavor to abide by them in every phase of his life.

1.1.4.4.2 *Relationship with professional organizations:* In order to inculcate a corporate life in his own professional colleagues, should join and advance the cause of all such organizations, the aims and objects of which are conducive to scientific, moral and cultural well-being of pharmacists and at the same time are in no way contrary to the code of Pharmaceutical ethics.

1.1.4.4.3 *Decorum and proprietary:* A pharmacist should always refrain from doing all such acts and deeds which are not in consonance with the decorum of pharmaceutical profession and are likely to bring discredit or upbraid to the profession or to him.

1.1.5 Pharmacist OATH

- I Swear by the code of Ethics of Pharmacy Council of India in relation to the community and shall act as an integral part of health care team.
- I shall uphold the laws and standards governing my profession.
- I shall strive to perfect and enlarge my knowledge to contribute to the advancement of pharmacy and public health.
- I shall follow the system, which I consider best for pharmaceutical care and counseling of patients.
- I shall endeavor to discover and manufacture drugs of quality to alleviate sufferings of humanity.
- I shall hold in confidence the knowledge gained about the patients in connection with professional practice and never divulge unless compelled to do so by the law.

- I shall associate with organizations having their objectives for betterment of the profession of Pharmacy and make contribution to carry out the work of those organizations.
- While I continue to keep this Oath inviolate, may it be granted to me to enjoy life and the practice of pharmacy respected by all, at all times!

Should I trespass and violate this oath, may the reverse be my lot!

1.2 COMMUNITY PHARMACY MANAGEMENT

The community pharmacy medicines management (CPMM) is a unique point with an objective to introduce a structured intervention process into the relationship study between the community pharmacist, the patient and the general practitioner. The study is designed as a randomized controlled trial (RCT).

1.2.1 Objectives

The *primary objectives* of the CPMM are:

(a) compare the proportion of the patients receiving appropriate treatment, as defined by currently available evidence and guidelines, between intervention and control groups at baseline and follow up.

(b) quantity "Health gain" by describing the change in patients overall health status after the intervention as defined by standard measures, both general and condition specific.

(c) conduct an economic evaluation of the medicines management intervention (including estimates of drug cost changes).

The *secondary objectives* are to

(a) describe the opinions of the stakeholders (patients, general practitioners and their staff and community pharmacists) of medicines management before and after its introduction.

(b) describe the role of over the counter (OTC) medicines in the overall patient management of this condition.

1.2.1.1 Function of materials management

1. Procurement of raw materials and other inputs required for production.
2. Maintaining stores and stock levels.

3.   Receiving and issuing of the materials.

4.   Transportation and material handling.

5.   Disposal of scrap and surplus material.

1.2.2 Legal Requirements

1.2.2.1 Legal requirements in purchasing

Law of contract, an agreement between to or more persons during business transaction. There must be lawful proposal by one party and lawful acceptance by the other party. So two parties can enter into the agreement. The form of agreement may be oral or in the form of writing.

1.2.2.2 Legal requirements involved in payment of price

There are three legal aspects involved in the payment of price:

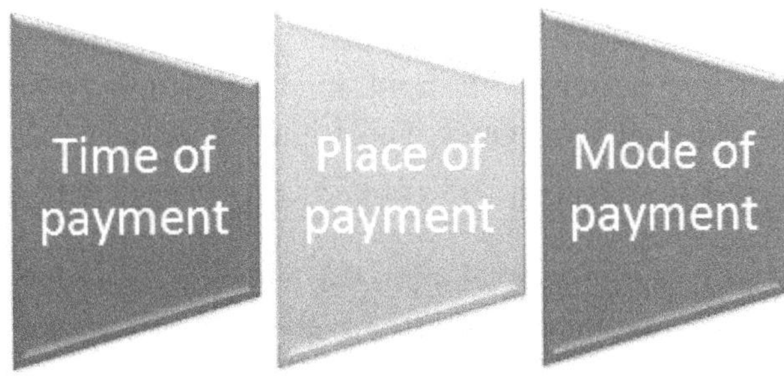

The buyer has to pay the due amount in time. If the buyer fails to inspect the goods within the reasonable time and find out whether all the items are in good condition and whether they confirm with their terms and conditions.

1.2.2.3 Legal requirements in pricing of bulk drugs

The drug price control order, 1987 authorities the central Government to fix the maximum sale price of the bulk drugs. While fixing prices of bulk drugs, the following points should be taken into consideration:

(i)   A past tax return of 14% on net worth.

(ii)   A return of 22% on capital employed.

(iii)   An internal return of 12% based on long term marginal costing in respect of new plant.

1.2.2.4 Legal requirements in pricing drug formulation

The drug price control order, 1987 authorized the central Government to fix the maximum sales price of drug formulation. It is based on the following formula:

$$RP = (MC+CC+PM+PC)X (1- MAPE/ 100) + ED$$

Where   RP = Retail price

MC = Material cost

CC = Conversion cost

PM = Cost of packaging materials

PC = Packaging charges

MAPE = Maximum allowable post-manufacturing expenses

ED = Excise duty

1.2.3 Staff Management

The right type of organization is selected, then it becomes necessary to fill in the various job positions with right kind of people, who can effectively performed their assigned activities. This is the management function of staffing.

1.2.3.1 Definition

The process of hiring and developing the required personnel to fill in various positions in the organization. It involves the scientific and systemic procurement, allocation, utilization, conversation and development of human resources.

The main objective of the staffing is to ensure the optimum utilization of human resources as well as to provide personal and social satisfaction to the employees.

1.2.3.2 Salient features of staffing

- Staffing is a function of management.
- It is a continuous function.
- It is a pervasive function.
- It is an integral part of the management process.
- It is a difficult function because it deals with human beings who have their own needs, emotions and aspiration.
- It is concerned with the human resources of an organization.

1.2.3.3 Importance of staffing

(i) Staffing helps to build up a healthy organization in which the job performance and satisfaction of every employee can be high.

(ii) Staffing injects life into the organization by providing right person for every job. The effectiveness of directing and control functions also depends upon staffing.

(iii) Employees in the organization are the most valuable asset of an organization. The quality of human assets largely determines the success and growth of the organization.

1.2.4 Material Management

Material Management is a basic function of the business that adds value directly to the product itself. Material Management is the planning, directing, controlling and coordinating the activities concerned with material and inventory requirements from the point of their inception to their introduction into the manufacturing process.

The two important aspects of material management includes:

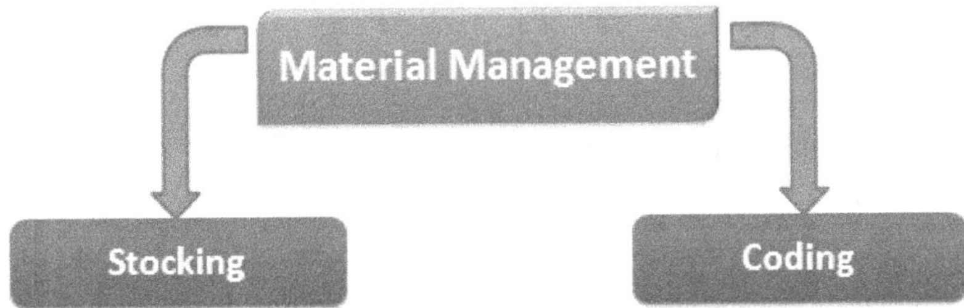

1.2.5 Stocking

The drug store should have adequate space for storage of drug with proper lighting, ventilation and temperature controls. Special locked storage space provided to meet the legal requirements for storage of narcotics, alcohol and prescribed drugs. The drugs are stored in such a way that they should not be damage due to high temperature. It is a fact that more than 70% of the capital of an enterprise is invested in stores.

1.2.5.1 Objectives of stocking

(a) Easy location of the items in store.

(b) Proper identification of items.

(c) Speedy issue of materials

(d) Efficient utilization of space.

(e) Reduction in needs of materials handling equipment.

1.2.5.2 Functions of stocking

(a) Receiving, handling and speedy issue of material.

(b) Custodian of goods in store against damage and pilferage.

(c) To establish regular supply of materials.

(d) Physical stocking and its checking.

(e) Efficient utilization of store space.

(f) To provide service to the organization in most economic way.

(g) Proper identification and easy location of items.

1.2.6 Arrangements of Drugs in Drug Store

The drugs may be arranged in the following manner:

1.2.6.1 According to manufacturer

The drugs are arranged in a drug store, manufacturer-wise for example, the drug manufactured by Glaxo (India) Ltd. are place in one cup-board and so on.

1.2.6.2 According to pharmacological action

The drugs may be arranged in order of their pharmacological action for example, all analgesics drugs are placed in one cupboard. All multivitamin preparations are kept in another cupboard and so on.

1.2.6.3 Alphabetical order

The drugs may also be arranged alphabetically. The drugs starting with letter "A" are placed in one row of the cupboard. Similarly with other drugs based on their first alphabet.

1.2.6.4 As per old stock and date of expiry

Drugs are stored in such a way that the older stock must be sold first, so that the old stock is stored in front row and the fresh stock is stored on the backside.

1.2.6.5 Location of stores for stocking

The location of stores in an enterprise should be at a place where handling, transporation and movement of the material is at a minimum level. If there is only single plant or many plants situated at the same area, then it is profitable to have one centralize store to serve all production operations.

The following are some of the advantages and disadvantages of centralized storing-

Advantages

  (a)   Economy in investments.

  (b)   Reduction in incidental expenses.

  (c)   Less storage of space.

  (d)   Less manpower required, due to which reduction in administrative costs.

  (e)   More bargaining power due to buying in bulk.

Disadvantages

  (a)   More materials handling operations.

  (b)   The chances of delay are likely to be more.

  (c)   More exposed to loss due to natural calamities like fire, rain, dust etc.

1.2.7 Coding or Codification

It is the process of assigning a code number or code symbol to a particular material for easy identification. Usually manufacturers, distributors and wholesalers have large merchandise in the stores. It is difficult to locate the items in the store unless some system is evolved to store them. There should be place for everything and it should be place at their right place. Therefore code numbers are allocated to various items to facilitate easy identification.

Advantages of codification

  (a)   It helps in easy identification of items.

  (b)   It helps in grouping the similar items together.

  (c)   The ambiguity in description of the materials can be avoided.

  (d)   The detailed description of the materials is minimized.

  (e)   It helps in avoiding duplication of items.

  (f)   It helps in physical counting.

  (g)   It helps in inspection of the materials.

  (h)   The coding helps in maintaining the secrecy of the items.

1.2.7.1 Methods of codification

The various methods employed for codification includes

1.2.7.1.1 *Alphabetical order method*

1.2.7.1.2 *Mnemonic method*

1.2.7.1.3 *Numerical method*

   (a)   Decimal system

   (b)   Block system

1.2.7.1.4 *Combination method or alphanumerical method*

1.2.7.1.5 *Location coding*

   (a)   Fixed location

   (b)   Random location

   (c)   Zonal location

1.2.7.1.1 *Alphabetical order method:* This method is also known as "Letter Code" system. In this system all items are on the code number alphabetically for example

Code "C" represents capsules

Code "T" represents tablets

1.2.7.1.2 *Mnemonic method:* In this method, coding letters assigned to each items so that they can be very easily identified for example "APC" represents aspirin, paracetamol and caffeine. The main disadvantage is that the items cannot be identified without refers *code index book*.

1.2.7.1.3 *Numerical method:* This method is also known as '*sequence system method*'. Under this method separate numbers are assigned to different classification of store items. The method has the following sub-systems-

(a) Block system

   In this method the numbers are reserved for specified items. Example let the number 10-50 is allotted to various types of tablets.

   10.1, 10.2, 10.3, 10.4, 10.5 represents antipyretic, analgesic, anti-inflammatory, decongestants and cold remedies respectively.

(b) Decimal system

   In this system, the numbers are assigned in such a way that each digit represents the separate name under same heading. example-

   Let the code for tablet is 10, then 10.1 (Paracetamol- antipyretic), 10.2 (Analgin-analgesic).

1.2.7.1.4 *Combination method:* In this method both mnemonic and numerical methods are combined to assign a code to different items of the store example Code number "CPC" is allotted from chloramphenicol capsules.

Code number "PAT 11" is allocated to paracetamol with analgin tablets.

This method is used when store items are quite large.

1.2.7.1.5 *Locating coding:* In a large organization, there are a large number of stores. The store rooms are divided in blocks and each block is identified by lateral block letter and longitudinal block letter. The location of items can be identified from ware-house number, block number, row number, rack number and shelf number etc.

Location of any item inside the store rooms can also be done in the following manner-

(a) Fixed location

In this method each and every group of items is allotted a fixed place inside the store according to either-

    (i)   Supplier wise

    (ii)   Item wise

    (iii)   According to the utility of the item.

(b) Random location

This is most widely used method in almost all kinds of retail shops but each group items are stored, in a particular shelf for its easy location.

(c) Zonal location

According to this system, available space is divided into different zones and each zone is allotted to different kinds of items. The zones can be named as-

    (i)   Bulk Zone

    (ii)   Reserve Stock Zone

    (iii)   Spare part Zone

    (iv)   Consumable Item zone

1.2.8 Space Layout

Plant layout is a method of allocating machines and equipments, various production processes and other necessary services involved in transformation process of a product with the available space of the factory, so as to perform various operations in the most efficient and convenient manner providing output of high quality and minimum cost.

Planning the layout of a plant is a continuous process as there are always chances of making improvements over the existing arrangements.

1.2.8.1 Objectives of an ideal plant layout

(i)   Material handling and transportation is minimized and efficiently controlled.

(ii) Work stations are designed suitable and properly.

(iii) Suitable spaces are allocated to production centers and service centers.

(iv) The movement made by workers is minimized.

(v)   Waiting time of the semi furnished product is minimized.

(vi) There are improved work methods and reduced production cycle means or times.

(vii) There is increased flexibility for changes in product design and for the future expansions.

(viii) A good layout permits materials to move through the plant at the desired speed with the lower cost.

1.2.8.2 Types of layout

There are mainly following types of layout-

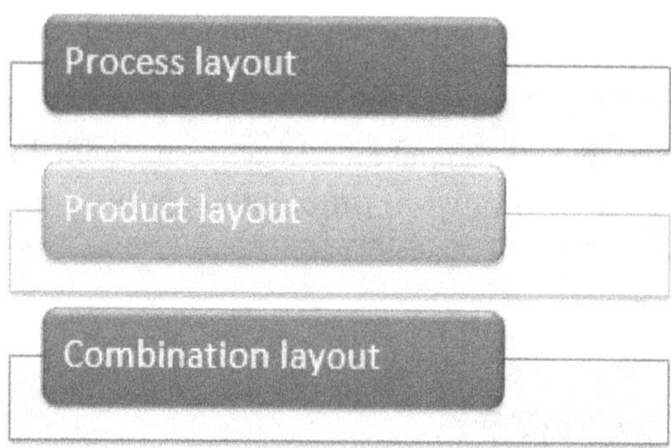

1.2.8.2.1 *Process layout*

It is also known as functional layout and is characterized by keeping similar machines or similar operation at one location. The arrangement of machines of a particular class doing a particular type of work or process as a separate department e.g. cutting machines may be placed under cutting department.

Advantages

  (i) Better machine utilization.

  (ii) Greater flexibility

  (iii) Better supervision which ultimately leads to better production.

  (iv) Less number of machines is needed involving reduced capital.

Disadvantages

- Functional Layout type may not be possible in the pharmaceutical and chemical industries, because a number of unit operations should be performed in sequence.

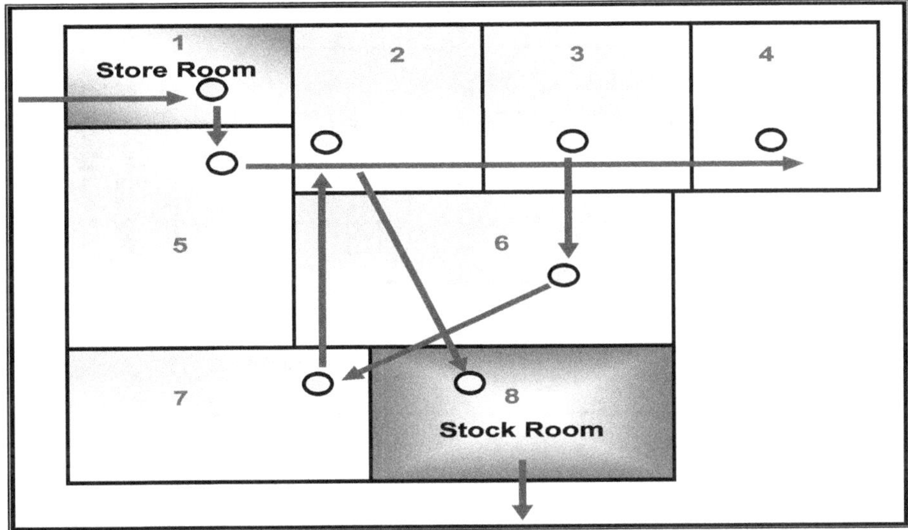

Fig. 1.3 Typical set up for Process Layout

1.2.8.2.2 *Product layout*

It is also called as ***straight line layout*** and according to the product manufactured. This set up of product layout is standardized in beginning. The product can be manufactured in large quantity by repetitive operation.

Advantages

  (i) Less space requirements for the same volume of production.

  (ii) Less in-process inventory.

  (iii) Smooth and continuous work flow.

(iv) Processing of work is quick and smooth.

(v) Cost of material handling can be reduced by using conveyors.

(vi) Manufacturing time is reduced and manufacturing cycle can be speeded up.

(vii) Floor space can be properly utilized.

This type of layout is **more suitable for the Pharmaceutical Industries.**

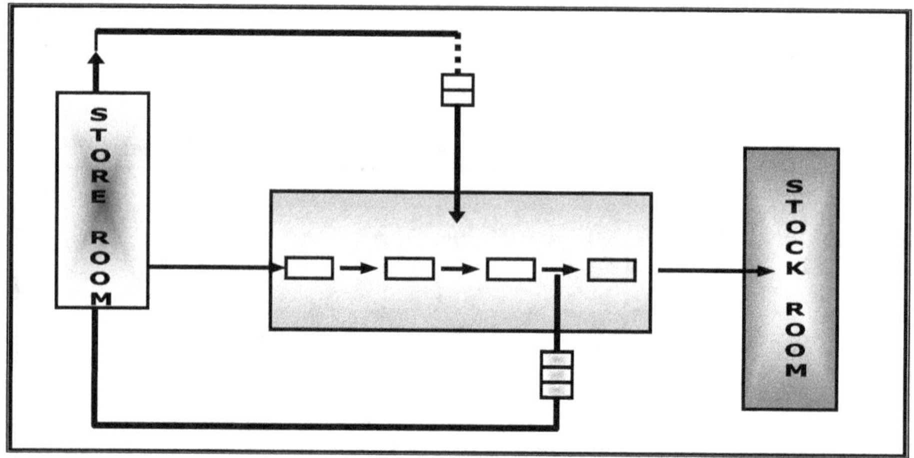

Fig. 1.4 Typical set up for Product layout

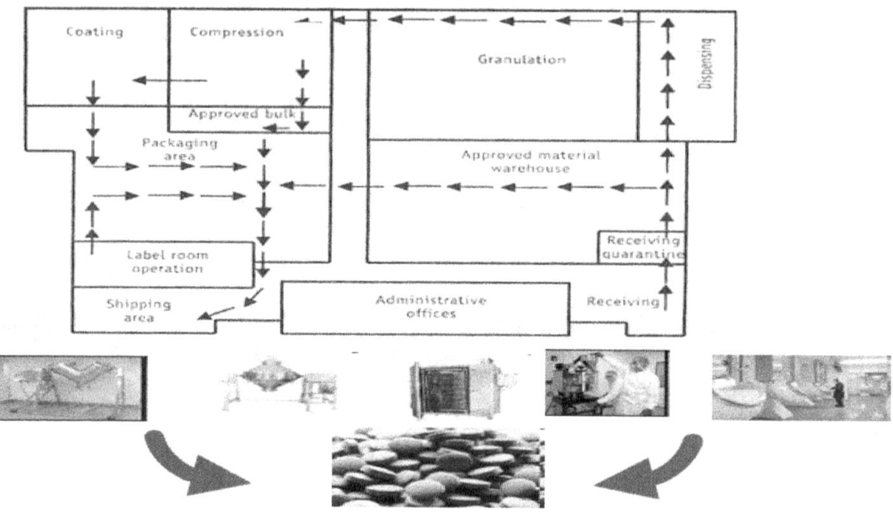

Fig. 1.5 Typical set up for Product layout for Tabletting Process
(Mixing, Granulation, Drying, Tablet Compression and Coating)

1.2.8.2.3 *Combination layout*

A combination of process and product layout combines the advantages of both types of layout. The layout should be efficient by keeping material handling at a minimum level. Suitable layout planning is required to keep the cost of product minimum.

1.2.9 Selection of Site

A plant is a place where men, materials and equipment are brought together for manufacturing procedures. The basic requirement for setting up a pharmaceutical industry is the availability of appropriate site.

1.2.9.1 Importance of plant location or site

The selection of appropriate location is important due to the following reasons-

1. Location of plant partially determines operating and capital cost. It determines the nature of investment costs to be incurred and also the levels of many operating costs.

2. Location fixes some of the physical factors of the overall plant design example heating and ventilation requirements, storage capacity of raw material taking into consideration their local availability.

3. Each prospective location implies a new allocation of capacity to respective market area.

4. Government some-times play an important role in the choice of the location keeping in view the national benefits.

1.2.10 Plant Location-Factors Influencing

The selection of a location for the construction of a pharmaceutical plant is a vital decision to be taken, because it determines the balancing of investment and profit. Hence the location of the plant has a strong influence on the success of an industrial venture. Primarily the plant should be located where the minimum cost of production and distribution can be achieved. But other factors such as room for expansion and general living conditions are also important. These factors may be described as follows:

1. Fundamental (Primary) Factors

2. Derived (Secondary factors)

1.2.10.1 Fundamental or primary factors

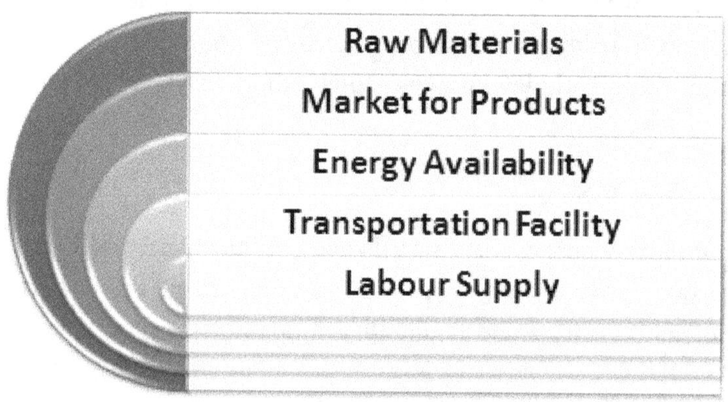

1.2.10.1.1 *Raw materials:* The availability of raw materials and cost of its transportation are the major determinants. Pharmaceutical industry uses the following types of raw materials: crude drugs, inorganic and organic chemicals etc. It would be economical to locate the plant nearer to the source of raw materials particularly when they are consumed in large volumes. If the raw materials are not readily available or a dangerous chemical, the freight charges and risk of dangers increase enormously. If raw materials are stable, other factors gain more importance over this factor.

1.2.10.1.2 *Market of products:* Market exercises a strong influence on the establishment of industries. When market is regional, the industry is located nearer to the market. The bulk drug industry is located in a place where drug formulation industries are located, since bulk drugs are the feed for the formulations and buyers are found nearby.

1.2.10.1.3 *Energy availability:* Fuel and power are the energy sources, which exert the same kind of influence as the raw materials. Now a days, electricity and diesel engines are developed and available widely. In many cases, plant produces power on their own for the smooth functioning of the industry. Therefore, it is possible to locate the industry remote to the power generation plants.

1.2.10.1.4 *Transportation facility:* Transportation is the lifeline of modern industry. Transport facilities are needed for bringing raw materials and sending the finished products. An industry tends to be localized at places, which have a developed means of transport such as railway, road and seaport. These facilities are normally available in metropolitan cities. Hence most of the industries are either located in such cities or in its vicinity.

1.2.10.1.5 *Labour supply:* Low wages and abundant labour help in localization of certain industries. However, pharmaceuticals and chemical plants require skilled labour, who are better paid and often highly mobile. Therefore, industries can be located away from the areas of labour concentration. Consideration should be given to prevailing pay rates, restrictions on number of hours per week, competing industries etc.

1.2.10.2 Derived (secondary) factors

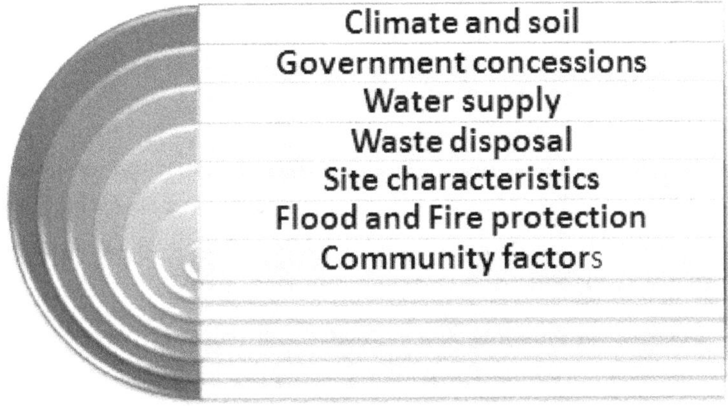

1.2.10.2.1 *Climate and soil:* Climate and soil is very important for industries depending on agriculture. In pharmaceutical industry, many operations are carried out in air-conditioned rooms, in dust free environments and under strict control and regulations depending upon the nature of formulation. Industries producing antibiotics are normally located in a place wherein the microbial contamination in environment is low and the ambient temperatures throughout the year are cool.

1.2.10.2.2 *Government concessions:* Government has been providing subsidies and tax concessions for the industries located in certain notified areas. These areas have been declared as industrially backward and the government offers incentives, namely cheaper power, tax concession etc.

1.2.10.2.3 *Water supply:* The processing industries use larger quantities of water for cooling, washing and steam generation and also as a raw material (liquid orals). The plant therefore must be located in a place where a dependable supply of water is available.

1.2.10.2.4 *Waste disposal:* In recent years, many legal restrictions have been imposed on the methods for disposing of waste materials from the processing industries. The site selected for a plant should have adequate capacity and facilities for correct waste disposal. Attention should also be given to potential requirements for additional waste treatment facilities.

1.2.10.2.5 *Site characteristics:* The topography of the land and soil structure must be considered, since either both may have a pronounced effect on construction costs. The cost of land, local building construction costs and living conditions are important. Future changes for expanding the plant facilities make it desirable or necessary.

1.2.10.2.6 *Flood and fire protection:* Many industries are located along large bodies of water and there are risks of flood or hurricane damage. Before choosing a plant site, the regional history of natural events of this kind should be examined. In case of major fire, assistance from the outside departments should be easily available.

1.2.10.2.7 *Community factors:* The character and facilities of a community can have quite an effect on the location of the plant. Cultural facilities of the community are important for sound growth. Churches, temples, libraries, schools, theaters and other similar groups, if active and dynamic, do much to make a community progressive.

1.2.11 Special provisions of Factory Premises: location

It is important to recognize that the pharmaceutical industry has some special requirement that need to be interpreted. The factory shall be located in a sanitary place remote from filthy surroundings. The factory shall be situated in place which:

(a) shall not be adjacent to an open sewage, drain or public lavatories.

(b) Shall not be adjacent to a factory, which produces disagreeable or obnoxious odours or fumes.

(c) Shall not be adjacent to a factory, which emits large quantities of soot, dust or smoke.

The factory shall not constitute undue danger to adjacent life and property. State laws and other related laws should be consulted. It becomes necessary for the entrepreneur to acquaint himself with all the legal controls, which are existing like Indian Factories Act, Drugs and Cosmetics Act and Rules etc. Checklist provides a useful means of evaluating a site location and other factors associated with its selection.

1.2.12   Use of Computers in Pharmacy

The computer has become one of a popular tool in all areas of science and technology. Right now computers and pharmacy go hand in hand. Today computers can provide the exchange of health information and services across geographic, time and social boundaries. Computers have revolutionized the way education is handled in the today's world. In medical education, computers are particularly useful because there is such a need for learning and presenting large amounts of data, getting and comparing accurate study and test results, and effectively monitoring patients.

With the proliferation of the Internet and the developments in computer technology and manufacturing, the ratio of price to performance of computers continues to decrease. This has resulted in the development of number of computer applications. The field of pharmacy has immensely benefited by the use of computer and will continue to benefit as the pharmacist's gain more familiarity with computers.

The complete field of pharmacy requires computers. Some of the important areas where computers are useful are ***new drug discovery, drug design, analysis, manufacturing of drugs and hospital pharmacy***. Other than these, computers helps pharmacist collaborate with other professionals, which is very essential in today's research work. It also provides solutions for time consuming manual task.

Various ***hardware and softwares have been developed without which drug discovery, designing, manufacturing and analyzing*** would become virtually impossible. Further development is still in progress which will make pharmacist's job easier. The more important fact is that they will enable us to discover new drugs for the complete care of dangerous of diseases like AIDS, cancer etc. and reduce the cost of production of drugs for diseases which are easily cured.

Computers are also useful for ***hospital pharmacist and in telemedicine***. A lot has been done and a still has to be done for improving the computer facilities for pharmacist.

1.2.12.1 Computer aided design of drugs

A further refinement of new drug design and production was provided by the process of computer-aided design (CAD). With the availability of powerful computers and sophisticated graphics software, it is possible for the medicinal chemist to design new molecules and evaluate their effectiveness.

1.2.12.2 Drug information services

Pharmaceutical companies are responsible for providing updated, relevant information on the efficacy, safety and quality of drugs to medical professionals and finally to patients. To fulfill this responsibility, they developed a drug information database system to manage various information generated during development of new products and after launch of the products. This system is incorporated into an on-line network system, and can be directly accessed by thousands of people all over the world.

1.2.12.3 Information system in pharmaceutical industries

An **information system** (IS) is any combination of information technology and people's activities using that technology to support operations, management, and decision-making.

Advanced pharmaceutical companies are realizing that the implementation of information management technologies in their operations can greatly enhance their chances for success by reducing their time-to-market and enhancing efficiency in their production runs.

Pharmacy informatics, also referred to as *pharmacoinformatics,* is one of the latest the application of computers to the storage, retrieval and analysis of drug and prescription information.

Pharmacy informaticists work with pharmacy information management systems that help the pharmacist make excellent decisions about patient drug therapies with respect to, medical insurance records, drug interactions, as well as prescription and patient information.

Pharmacy informatics can be thought of as a sub-domain of the larger professional discipline of health informatics. Some definitions of pharmacy informatics reflect this relationship to health informatics. For example, the Health Information Management Systems Society (HIMSS) defines pharmacy informatics as, "the scientific field that focuses on medication-related data and knowledge within the continuum of healthcare systems - including its acquisition, storage, analysis, use and dissemination - in the delivery of optimal medication-related patient care and health outcomes" (HIMSS October 2006).

PRESCRIPTION AND INVENTORY CONTROL

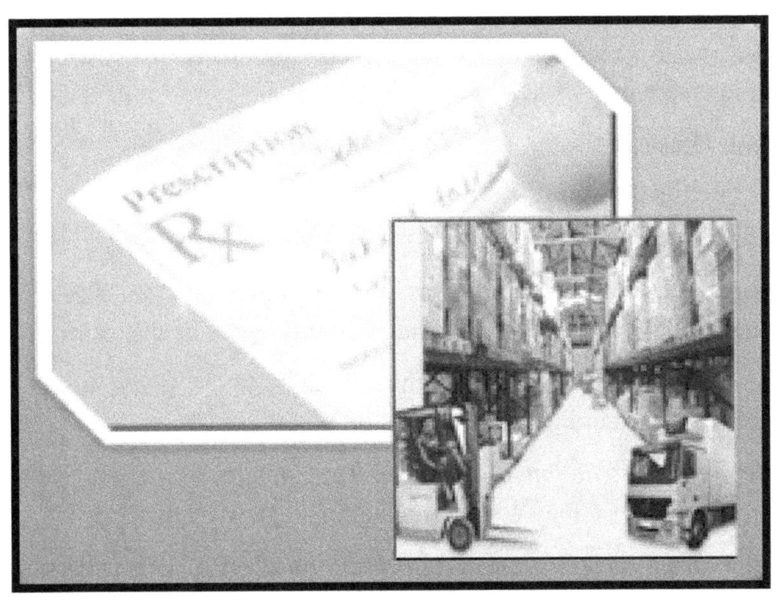

2.1 PRESCRIPTION

It is a written order from a registered medical practitioner or other practitioners such as dentists etc. to a pharmacist to compound and dispense a specific medication for the patient.

2.1.1 Parts of Prescription

Prescriptions are generally written on a typical format which is usually kept as Writing Pads. A typical format of prescription consists of following parts:

(a) *Date-* It helps a pharmacist to find out the date of prescribing and date of presentation for filling the prescription.

(b) *Name, age, sex and address of the patient-* Name, age and sex of the patient must be written on the prescription because it serves to identify the prescription.

(c) *Superscription-* It is represented by the symbol "*Rx*" which is written before writing the prescription. It is a latin word which means "*you take*". In olden days, the symbol was considered to be originated from the sign of Jupiter, God of healing. This symbol was employed in requesting God for quick recovery of the patient.

(d) *Inscription-* This is the main part of the prescription order. It contains the names and quantities of the prescribed ingredients. It is divided into the following parts

    (a) Base

    (b) Adjunct and

    (c) Vehicle

(e) *Subscription-* This comprises the direction to the pharmacist for preparing the prescription and number of doses to be dispensed.

(f) *Signature-* This consists of the direction to be given to the patient regarding the administration of the drug.

(g) *Renewal Instructions-* the prescriber indicate on every prescription order, whether it may be renewed and if so, how many times.

(h) *Signature, Address and registration number of the prescriber-* The prescription must bear the signature of the prescriber along with its registration number and address.

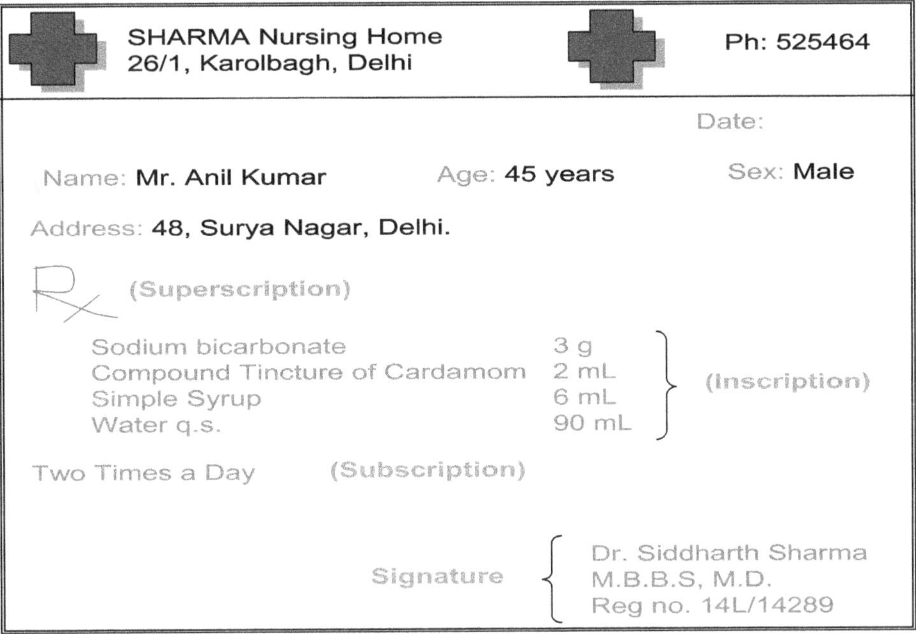

Fig. 2.1 Format of a Prescription.

2.1.2 Legality and Identification of Medication

A medication-related problem is an event or situation involving drug therapy that negatively interferes with a patient's health. Medication-related problems can be categorized as:

(a) Untreated conditions

The patient has a medical condition that requires drug therapy but is not receiving a drug for that condition.

(b) Drug use without indication

The patient is taking a medication for no medically valid condition or reason.

(c) Improper drug selection

The patient's medical condition is being treated with the wrong drug or a drug that is not the most appropriate for the special needs of the patient.

(d) Subtherapeutic dosage

The patient has a medical problem that is being treated with too little of the correct medication.

(e) Overdosage

The patient has a medical problem that is being treated with too much of the correct medication.

(f) Adverse drug reactions (ADRs)

The patient has a medical condition that is the result of an adverse drug reaction or adverse effect. In the case of older adults, ADRs contribute to already existing geriatric problems such as urinary incontinence, constipation, and weight loss.

(g) Drug interactions

The patient has a medical condition that is the result of a drug interacting negatively with another drug or food.

(h) Failure to receive medication

The patient has a medical condition that is the result of not receiving a medication due to economic, psychological, sociological, or pharmaceutical reasons.

2.1.2.1 Drug interactions incompatibility

Drug Interactions are said to occur when the pharmacologic activity of a drug is altered by the concomitant use of another drug or by presence of food, drink or environmental chemicals.

The drug whose activity is affected by such interaction is called as the *object drug* and the agent which is precipitates such interaction is referred as *precipitant.* Most interactions are specific types of adverse reactions with altered efficacy of the drug. For example, Enhancement of activity of penicillin when administered with probenecid.

2.1.2.2 Types of interactions

2.1.2.2.1 *Pharmacokinetic interactions* are those in which the absorption, distribution, metabolism and/or excretion (ADME) of the object drug are altered by the precipitant.

(a) Interactions affecting absorption of drugs

Altered absorption after oral administration is very common. The interaction may result in a change in the rate of absorption (an increase or decrease), a change in the amount of drug absorbed or both. In general, drugs that are not absorbed completely are more susceptible to changes in GI absorption.

(b) Interactions affecting distribution of drugs

Significant interactions results due to competition between drugs for binding to proteins or tissues and displacement of one drug by the other. Greater Risk of interactions exists when the displaced drug is highly protein bound (more than 95 %), has a small volume of distribution and has a narrow therapeutic index. For example, Warfarin, phenytoin etc.

(c) Interactions affecting metabolism of drugs

The most important and the most common cause of pharmacokinetic interactions is alterations in the rate of biotransformation of drugs. Major problem arises when one drug either induces or inhibits the metabolism of another drug. The influence of enzymes inducers and inhibitors become more pronounced when drugs susceptible to first-pass hepatic metabolism are given concurrently.

(d) Interactions affecting excretion of drugs

Excretion pattern can be affected by alterations in glomerular filtration rate (GFR), renal blood flow, passive and active tubular secretion and urine pH. An interesting pharmacokinetic interaction that results due to the pharmacodynamic drug effect is between thiazide diuretics and lithium. List of some of the important pharmacokinetic interactions are shown in Table 2.1

Table 2.1 Pharmacokinetic Interactions.

Object drug(s)	Precipitant drug(s)	Influence on object drug(s)
ABSORPTION INTERACTIONS		
1. Complexation and Adsorption		
Tetracycline, penicillin	Antacids, food and mineral supplements containing aluminum, magnesium, iron, zinc and calcium ions.	Formation of poorly soluble and unabsorbable complex with such heavy metal ions
Ciprofloxacin, norfloxacin	Antacids containing aluminum, magnesium and calcium.	Reduced absorption
2. Alteration of GI pH		
Sulphonamides, aspirin	Antacids	Enhanced dissolution
Ferrous sulphate	Sodium bicarbonate, calcium carbonate	Decreased dissolution

Table 2.1 *Contd...*

METABOLISM INTERACTIONS		
1. Enzyme Induction		
Corticosteroids, oral contraceptives, phenytoin	Barbiturates	Decreased plasma levels
Corticosteroids, oral contraceptives, phenytoin	Phenytoin	Decreased plasma levels
2. Enzyme Inhibition		
Tyramine rich food (cheese, liver)	MAO Inhibitors (phenelzine)	Potentially fatal risk of hypertensive crisis.
Folic acid	Phenytoin	Decreased absorption of folic acid
3. Alteration of gut motility		
Aspirin, diazepam, levodopa, lithium carbonate	Metoclopramide	Rapid gastric emptying
Levodopa, lithium carbonate	Anticholinergics	Delayed gastric emptying
DISTRIBUTION INTERACTIONS		
1. Competitive displacement interactions		
Anticoagulants (warfarin)	Phenyl butazone, chloral hydrate	Increased clotting time
Phenytoin	Valporic acid	Phenytoin toxicity
Tolbutamide	Sulfonamides	Increased hypoglycemic effect
EXCRETION INTERACTIONS		
1. Changes in active tubular secretion		
Penicillin, PAS, Dapsone, Nalidixic acid	Probenecid acid	Risk of toxic reactions
Ranitidine, Procainamide	Cimetidine (base)	Risk of toxicity
2. Changes in Urine pH		
Amphetamine, Tertracycline	Anatacids, Thiazides	Increased passive reabsorption of basic drugs
3.Changes in renal blood flow		
Lithium	NSAIDs (Non steroidal anti-inflammatory drugs)	Decreased renal clearance of lithium, risk of toxicity

2.1.2.2.2 *Pharmacodynamic interactions* are those in which the activity of the object drug at its site of action is altered by the precipitant. Such interactions may be direct or indirect.

(a) **Direct pharmacodynamic interaction** is the one in which drugs having similar or opposing pharmacological effects are used concurrently. The three consequences of direct interactions are-

   (i) *Antagonism*: The interacting drugs have opposing action example acetyl choline and noradrenaline have opposing side effects on heart rate.

   (ii) *Addition or summation*: The interacting drugs have similar actions and the resultant effect is the sum of individual drug responses. For example, CNS depressants like sedatives, hypnotics etc.

   (iii) *Synergism*: It is the enhancement of action of one drug by another. For example, Alcohol enhances the analgesic activity of aspirin.

(b) **Indirect pharmacodynamic interactions** are the situations in which both the object and the precipitant drugs have unrelated effects but the latter in some way alters the effects of the former. For example, Salicylates decreases the activity of platelets to aggregate thus impairing the homeostasis if warfarin induced bleeding occurs.

2.2 INVENTORY CONTROL

2.2.1 Introduction

Inventory is a detailed list of those movable items which are necessary to manufacture a product and to maintain the equipments and machinery in good working order. The quantity and value of every item is also mentioned in the list.

It is defined as a systemic control over maintenance of stock in the store department.

Inventory means all the raw materials, spare parts, tools, maintenance consumables, fuels, lubricants, semi-processed materials and finished goods etc.

On an average about *30 % of total working capital* is spent on inventories. Therefore, it is very important that for smooth working of the business organization, a sound inventory should be maintained. It should neither be excessive nor inadequate but it should be of optimum level.

Inventory control is an effective way to keep control over losses from misappropriation, damage, deterioration, evaporation and carelessness. This is necessary because investment in materials constitutes a major portion of the cost of production. In broader terms inventory control is about knowing and verifying, what you have and should have? Where it is? Where it should be? Knowing when to replenish items appropriate to function.

Inventory management may be defined as a scientific method of finding out how much stock should be maintained in order to meet the production demands and be able to provide right type of material at right time, in right quantities and at competitive prices. A well managed inventory can exert considerable financial leverage and inventory reduction. Such a conversation of cash is needed for investing in more profitable ventures and also helps in reducing borrowing. The words "inventory control" and "inventory management" are used interchangeably.

To satisfy the needs of inventory control and achieve reduction requires appropriate capture and management of inventory data, and where possible synchronization of production to customer demand.

2.2.2 Objectives of Inventory Control

The main objectives of inventory control are:

1. To maintain sufficient inventory so as to avoid production held up which leads to customer dissatisfaction loss of revenue and increase in cost.

2. Only the required quantities of material will be stocked in the stores and there is no need to keep the material in excess, which will lead to blockage of money.

3. With proper control of inventories the materials can be purchased well in advanced by inviting the tenders/quotations.

4. During stock period the number of workers can be reduced whereas in boom periods the man power can be increased, thus money can be saved.

5. With proper planning of production the wastage and surplus can be reduced, because now a day tastes of people are changing so materials should be cautiously stored to prevent the wastage of material and money.

6. Production will have to be done according to the time of demand. This will only be possible if the raw materials required for production are available in the stores.

7. Having control over the inventories the theft of small but costly items can be checked.

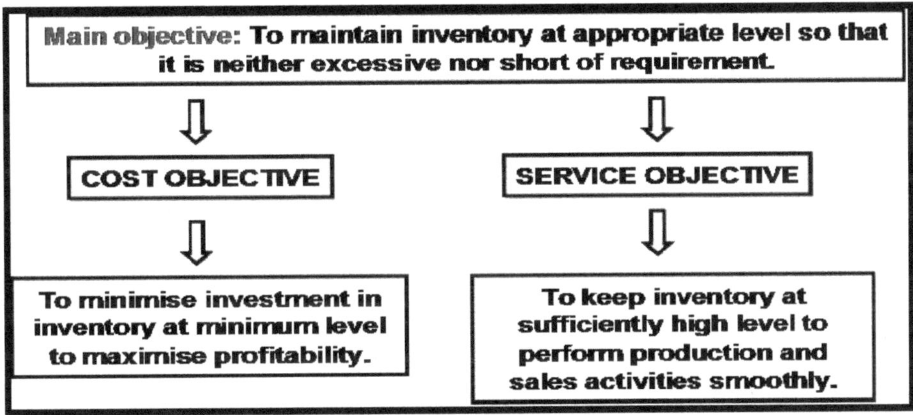

Fig. 2.2 Objectives Involved with Inventory Process.

2.2.3 Functions of Inventory Control

1. Persons, machines and materials are properly utilized.

2. To assess the material requirement systematically.

3. Wastage of materials and theft of materials can be checked.

4. The production can be supplied to the consumers at a short notice as and when the demand is received.

5. To obtain and supply the required quantity of materials at the lowest cost of proper time.

6. To keep the inventories as low as possible, this leads to consistent price in market conditions.

7. To maintain proper records to assess the stock position of the materials.

2.2.4 Types of Inventories

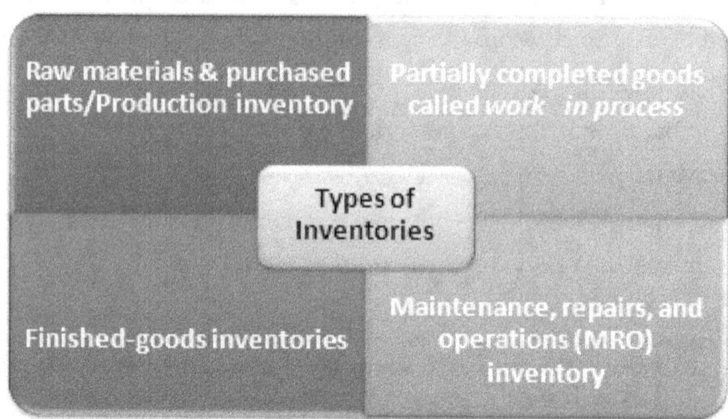

2.2.5 Techniques of Inventory Control

The following techniques are commonly used to control the inventory-

- ABC analysis
- VED analysis
- Perpetual inventory control system
- Lead time method
- Safety stock method
- Minimum and maximum stock levels
- Economic order quantity (EOQ) method
- HML classification
- FSN classification
- SDE classification

2.2.5.1 ABC analysis or ABC method

ABC stands for always better control. This is a selective analysis based on annual inventory value. For better and economical control of items in inventory, the items should be classified according to their significance or priority for re-ordering.

The inventory of high value items is to be controlled carefully due to high turnover and heavy investments. For the lower value items, the cost of inventory management is significant and should be controlled because it may be more than the possible inventory savings.

According to this approach, the items are classified into three main categories:

(a) A-class

(b) B-class

(c) C-class

(a) ***Group A items***: It consists of costly items which are 10 to 20 % of the total items, but has more than 50 % of total value of goods. It needs maximum follow up and require no safety stocks.

(b) ***Group B items***: It covers 20 % of the total inventories and represents 30 % of total value of stores and also requires low safety stocks.

(c) ***Group C items***: It covers 70 % of the total inventories and consumes 10 % of total expenditure of inventories.

Table 2.2   Major Characteristics of various categories of ABC approach.

Class A	Class B	Class C
Very strict control	Moderate Control	Loose control
No/very low safety stocks	Low safety stocks	Highly safety stocks
Maximum follow up	Periodic follow up	Follow up in exceptional case
Frequent ordering/ weekly delivery	Once in three months	Bulk ordering once in six months

Advantages

1. It ensures better control over costly items.
2. It helps in maintaining the stock in a better approach.
3. It helps in reducing the storage costs.
4. It helps in developing scientific method of controlling inventories.

Disadvantages

1. B & C Categories can often get neglected and pile in huge stocks or susceptible to loss and slackness in record control.

2.2.5.2 VED analysis

VED stands for **"*vital essential and desirable analysis*"**. This system is based on the utility of the materials. Based on the usage, the items/ materials are divided into three categories:

(a) *Vital:* Vital materials are the most essential items for production. Without these materials, production is stopped for a period of several days.

(b) *Essential:* These are the items which are very essential for production. Without this material, production is stopped only for a few hours or a day.

(c) *Desirable:* These items are needed by any organization but do not cost any effect on its performance.

For example, Acetyl salicylic acid is available as Disprin tablets, Anacin tablets and APC tablets. Disprin tablets have high demand followed by others. Hence, Disprin tablets are vital, Anacin as essential and APC comes under desirable category.

2.2.5.3   Perpetual inventory control systems

Proper examination with regard to receipts, issue and balance of materials in hand is done every time when the stock is handled and moreover the entire stock is rechecked. The major characteristics of perpetual inventory control system includes-

- An inventory accounting system that monitors inventory constantly.

- Reflecting the physical movement of stocks and their current balances.

- Just like keeping track of how much inventory has been sold at point of sale by recording selling price and type of item sold. For example, A bar code scanning system.

- A separate account in the subsidiary ledger is maintained for each good in stock, and the account is updated each time a quantity is added or taken out.

- Each column gives information on quantity, unit cost, and total cost.

The perpetual inventory system consist of-

- (a)   Bin card
- (b)   Stores ledger
- (c)   Continuous stock-taking.

- **(a)** *Bin card:* Record of all items of materials and goods in the store is recorded in this document. It shows the quantities of each material received, issued and in stock. A typical format of the bin card is shown in Figure 2.3.

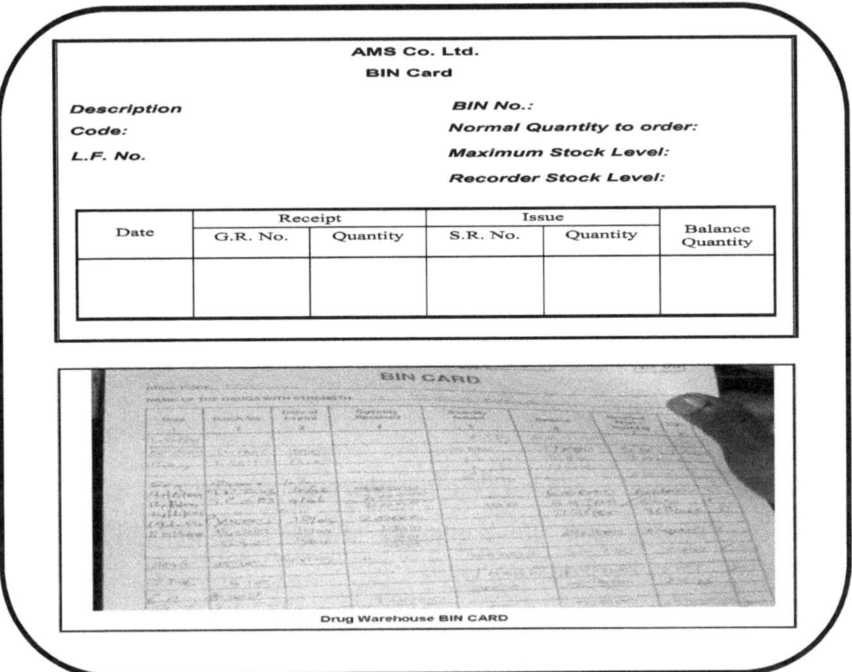

Fig. 2.3 Bin Card.

(b) *Store ledger:* It is maintained by cost accounting department.

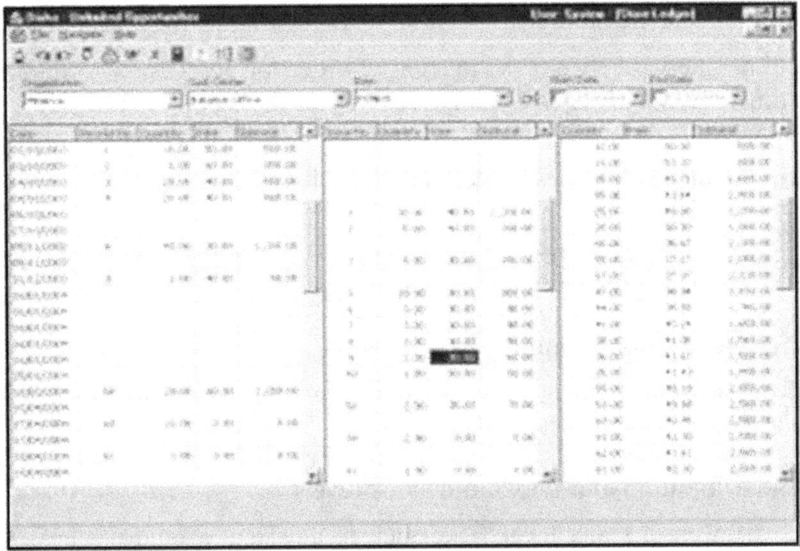

Fig. 2.4 Store Ledger (Cost Accounting Department).

Advantages

- Detection & rectification of errors.
- Checking of store items.
- Helps in loss accounts, balance sheet.
- Over & under stocking is avoided.
- High degree of control.
- Improves the quality of the physical stock taking.
- Maintain higher work standards.
- Unauthorized changes in procedures are detected and production hold-ups, a common issue in periodic stocktaking is eliminated.

Disadvantages

- Time-consuming.
- Manpower needed as it involves more frequent stocktaking.

(c) ***Continuous stock taking-*** Periodically limited numbers of items are checked and data is compared.

Advantages

(a) It helps to detect clerical errors.
(b) It helps in preparation of profit and loss account.
(c) Capital investment in materials will be under control.
(d) It makes available correct stocks figure.

2.2.5.4 Lead time method

The time interval between the placing of order for purchase of certain items to the time, the materials is actually received in the stores. It has two important components:

(a) ***Administrative/ servicing lead time-*** It is taken by the organization for placing the order.
(b) ***Supplier lead time-*** The time gap between the placements of order to the receipt of goods in the store is known as suppliers lead time.

2.2.5.5 Safety stock method

A firm has to keep adequate stock as well as ordinary stock. Overstocking of goods is known as "*Safety stocks*".

2.2.5.6 Minimum and maximum stock levels

(a) **Minimum stock level**: The stock of any item should not be allowed to fall below the lower limit. This is known as "*minimum stock level*". If the items are out of stock, it is not possible to supply the materials in time to the consumers. So minimum stock level should be maintained. This level is determined by-

   (i)   Rate of consumption.
   (ii) Recorder level.
   (iii) Time taken to receive fresh supplies from the producers.

(b)   Maximum stock level: The stock of any item should not be allowed to rise beyond the upper limit called as *"maximum stock level"*. If the stock is beyond the upper limit, then company has to invest large amounts. This level is determined by

   (i)   Rate of consumption.
   (ii) Re-order level.
   (iii) Time taken to receive fresh supplies.
   (iv) Amount of capital needed.
   (v)   Market trend.
   (vi) Nature of the material.

2.2.5.7 Economic order quantity (EOQ) method

The EOQ is the level of inventory and reorder quantity at which the combined costs of purchasing and carrying inventory are at a minimum. It is used to find out how much of the goods are to be ordered. The correct quantity to be ordered is determined by considering the following factors;

   (a) ordering cost and
   (b) The inventory carrying cost.

2.2.5.7.1 *Methods of determination of EOQ*

   1. *Tabular column method*: The purchasing details are written in a tabular column, as shown in Figure 2.5.

		Tabular Column Method		
SNo.	No. of orders per year	Annual ordering Cost (Rs.)	Annual Inventory Carrying Cost (Rs.)	Total Annual cost (Rs.)
1	12	1200	500	1700
2	6	600	1000	1600

Total Annual Cost = Annual Ordering Cost + Annual Inventory Carrying Cost

Fig. 2.5 Tabular Column Method.

2. *Algebric method*

EOQ can also be determined by using the following formula

$$EOQ = \sqrt{\frac{2\ (\text{Annual usage in units})\ (\text{Order cost})}{(\text{Annual carrying cost per unit})}}$$

Applications

1. EOQ formula is a good technique for calculating the economical lot size for ordering.

2. EOQ relationship also shows, a general way, how much inventories should be increased, if the sales of the product is increased by 20 %.

3. According to EOQ formula, the maximum inventory would be the square root of 20.

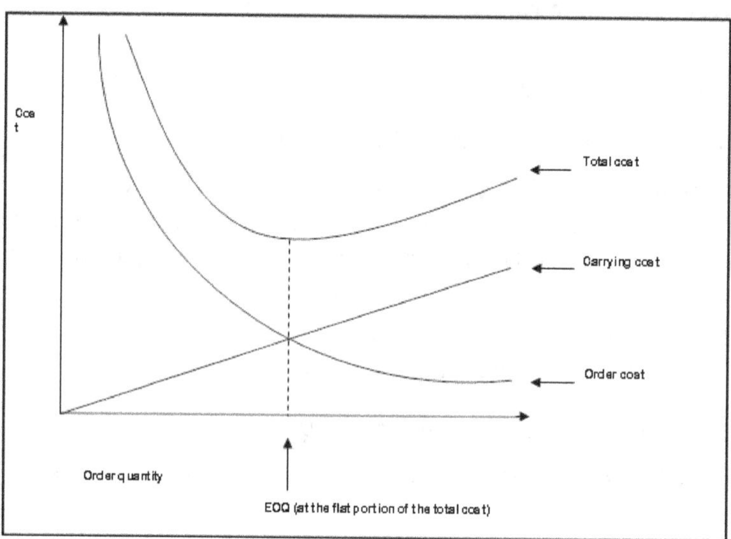

Fig. 2.6 Graphical Representation of Determination of EOQ Method.

2.2.5.7.2 *Costs involved in EOQ*

The economic lot size depends upon two types of cost:

1. **Procurement cost**: The procurement cost consists of expenditure concerned with the following:

   - Receiving quotations.
   - Processing purchase requisition.

- Follow-up and expediting the purchase order.
- Receiving items and inspecting the items.
- Processing vendor's invoice.

    Procurement cost decreases as the order quantity increases, because fewer orders are possible.

2. **Carrying cost**: It consists of expenditure connected with the following:
   - Interest on capital investment.
   - Cost of storage facility, up-keep of materials, record keeping etc.
   - Cost involving deterioration and obsolescence.
   - Cost of insurance, property tax etc.

     Carrying cost varies with quantity ordered. If smaller is the order, carrying cost is reduced. In such cases, number of orders increase (i.e. procurement cost).

     EOQ model provides a level of inventory at which the combined costs of procuring and carrying inventory are at minimum.

Total Inventory cost= Procurement cost+ Carrying cost

Advantages

- It minimizes ordering and holding cost while avoiding stock out cost.
- It gives a useful approximation for keeping some extra inventory on hand.

Limitations

- Include assumption of stable, continuation use pattern and consistent pricing.
- Assumes storage space is unlimited.
- Assumes ordering costs are accurately known.
- Assumes carrying costs are accurately known.
- Sometimes, EOQ quantities may not balance with quantities of all items needed for a lot size. Several other items are also needed simultaneously. In such cases, the inventory costs increases.
- It is not time-phased and assumes that some inventory should be replenished as soon as it is depleted.

- EOQ may not be applicable when the demands are irregular or where there is possibility of price rise.
- The Inventory holding cost and the ordering costs cannot be identified or calculated accurately.
- Computer systems or stock record cards must be maintained up to date on the items.
- If the minimum direct order quantity exceeds the EOQ by considerable amount, then direct order quantity must be considered.
- Set-up cost is also important factor. In such cases, a technique called LIMIT (Lot-size Inventory Management Interpolation Technique) can be used.

2.2.5.8 HML classification

HML stands for *high, medium and low*. This method is similar to ABC method, which is based on annual value of consumption. The items should be listed in decreasing order of unit value and management may fix limits for deciding the three categories.

2.2.5.9 FSN classification

FSN stands for *fast moving, slow moving and non-moving*. FSN classification comes in handy when obsolescence is to be controlled. There may be a change in technology or a change in the specification or an item is no longer in use. In such cases, FSN classification is made and information should be displayed prominently enabling managers to act on it in the best interest of the organization.

2.2.5.10 SDE classification

SDE stands for *scarce (longer lead time), difficult (long lead time) and easy (reasonably lead time)*. If an item is scarce and in A-category then the normal procedure cannot be applied for the stocking. These items may be:

(a) Imported.

(b) Not easily available in the market.

(c) Very difficult to manufacturer.

If an item is easy to obtain and an A-item, then care is required as for treatment of the A-item. But if it is C-item, inventory controller really does not have to bother very much.

2.2.6 Re-order Quantity Level

- Re-order quantity level is the level of purchasing where a new order of supply of material is to be placed.

- Re-order point are usually based on the usage during the time to re-order and receive materials and believed to reach when the inventory on hand and quantities are equal to the lead time.

- There are several factors that determine appropriate order point.

   - Delivery time stock (inventory needed during lead time)

   - Safety Stock (minimum level of inventory that acts as a protection against shortage due to high demand)

Therefore, the re-order point:

Ordering point or re-order level = Maximum daily or weekly or monthly usage × Lead time + Safety stock

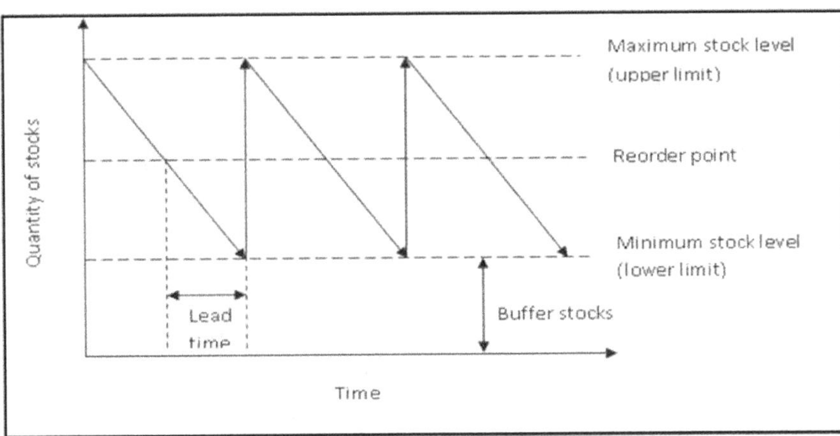

Fig. 2.7 Graphical Representation showing Determination of Ordering Point.

- It is fixed between minimum level and maximum level.

- Minimum level shows quantity which need to be maintain all the time. Less stock means that work will be stop due to shortage of the material due to high demand.

Factors those are important while fixing minimum stock level is

1. *Lead time*

The time taken in processing the order and then executing.

2. *Rate of consumption*

It is average consumption of material in factory.

3. *Nature of the materials*

When materials required only against the special order of customer, no minimum stocks are needed.

- Maximum level shows the quantity of material beyond the stocks required.

- If the quantity exceeds the maximum level, it will cause overstocking that cause increasing material cost, more working capital, more spaces needed for the purpose of storing the material and more wastage and high chances of losses from obsolescence occur.

2.2.7 Safety Stocks

- It is important as it is a buffer to meet some unexpected increase in the usage of the materials.

- It is also important in preventing stock-out from happen.

- Stock-out will cause

    - production disruption.

    - failure of the firm in competition with others as it cannot provide customer services and cannot fulfill the customer needs and requirements.

- Low quantity of safety stocks will lead to frequent occurrence of stock-out that result in large opportunity cost.

- While large quantity of safety stock will lead to higher carrying cost of the materials.

Advantages

- Avoid zero-stock level.

- Able compensate the errors in forecasting techniques.

Disadvantages

- Increases storage costs.

- Do not account for unusual delays in delivery.

- Require the need for rechecking the reorder quantity level periodically to allow for a change in usage rate.

2.2.8 Just-in-time Inventory Control

- A technique for inventory control that emphasizes on having the required materials or items arrived just as they are needed in the production process. Pharmaceutical organization need to have access to the right materials at the right place and time.

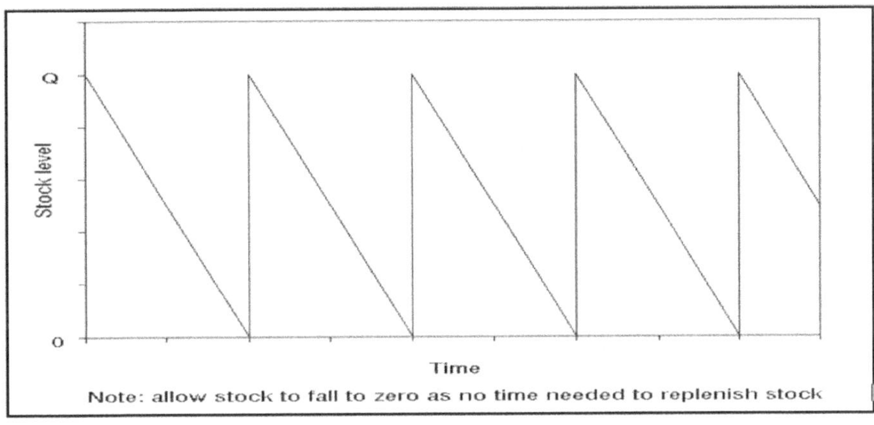

Fig. 2.8 Graphical Representation to Determine Safety Stock.

Advantages

- Holding backup materials in inventory for a long period of time is not needed.

- Holding cost can be kept at minimum level.

- Storage space is saved.

Disadvantages

- This technique is only practical for easily available materials.
- Delay in the arrival of materials can halt the production line.
- No significant amount of inventory to cover mistakes in forecasting.

2.2.9 Modern Inventory Control Systems

2.2.9.1 Vendor managed inventory (VMI)

VMI is the latest concept in which the manufacturer (vendor) creates orders for their distributors or customers based on the demands or requests made by the distributors or customers. Inventory levels, fill rates and costs are determined by an agreement between the vendor and customer. Electronic Data Interchange (EDI) act as the mean of communication between the two parties. Based on the information, the vendor will decide when to generate the purchase order.

Advantages

Vendors and Supplier/Distributor

- Reduces human data entry errors.
- A true partnership is formed.

Vendors

- Better insight in customer demand.
- Improved, more direct communication with customers. Improved market analysis.
- A reduction in distributor returns due to improved ordering.

Suppliers

- Reduced replenishment times and lower inventory costs.
- Increased sales through reduced stock outs.
- Vendor assistance with category management.

End-users

- Increased service level.
- Reduced stock-outs.

Disadvantages

- Success of VMI initiative depends on the strength of relationship between the vendors and retailers.
- Increased dependency between the parties and increased switching costs.
- Lack of trust to exchange data can result in ineffective implementation of inventory invisibility and inventory imbalance.
- Most of the benefits are for the end client and for the selling party, while the vendor does much of the work.

2.2.9.2 Radiofrequency identification (RFID) microchips

RFID allows a business to identify individual products and components, and to track them throughout the supply chain from production to point-of-sale. RFID is a technology that uses radio waves for communication between a tag (data carrier or RF transponder) and a reading device. The reader (or interrogator) is usually capable of reading data from and writing data to the tag. An RFID tag is a tiny microchip, plus a small aerial, which can contain a range of digital information about a particular item.

Advantages of RFID

- Tags can be read remotely, often at a distance of several metres.
- Several tags can be read at once.
- Tags can be given unique identification codes, so that individual products can be tracked.

- To prevent over-stocking or under-stocking a product or component for stock security, by positioning tag-readers at points of high risk, such as exits, and causing them to trigger alarms.

Disadvantages of RFID

- It imposes higher cost in products.

2.2.9.3 Material requirement planning (MRP)

It is a computational technique that converts the master-schedule of production into a detailed schedule for the materials and components used in the production. It determines the quantity of materials and the date on which these are needed for each phase of production.

Advantages

- It is applicable to inventory type, raw materials, components and work-in-progress.
- It is useful when there is a sudden change in demand in the market or sudden change in quantity or date.
- It is effective in minimizing unnecessary inventory investment.
- It ensures improved customer service.

Disadvantages

- In this system, procurement costs are high because each item is processed separately.
- Close monitoring of material stocks is essential.

2.3   INVENTORY CONTROL IN WAREHOUSES

2.3.1 Introduction

Warehouse is a store house for goods in which store items are to be kept which are in continuing requirement within virtually any supply chain. In warehouses the pre as well as post production items are being stored. Warehouse and inventory control business need to determine if their facilities can match the demands.

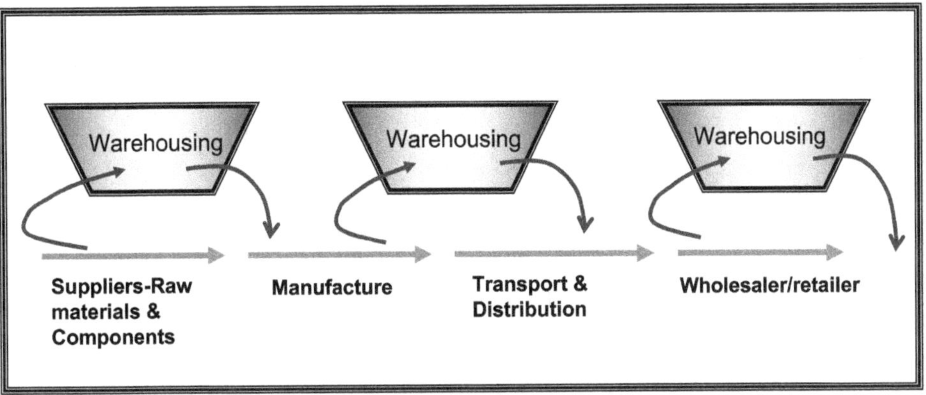

Fig. 2.9 Various Processes Involving Warehousing.

Now a days lot of efforts are being made to improve those processes which involve paper based and manual data collection. These are error prone and slow compared with the automatic or semiautomatic data capture. For example, Speeding up and improving the accuracy of a goods receipt process may allow the inventory to be better controlled.

2.3.2 Principle Features of Traditional Warehouse Activity

1. Receiving and putting away.

2. Picking and packaging.

3. Shipping.

4. Inventory control.

2.3.2.1 Receiving and putting away

Where information concerning incoming items to a warehouse is in written or human readable form and requires manual transcription and/or key-board entry into the warehouse computer system is likely to below.

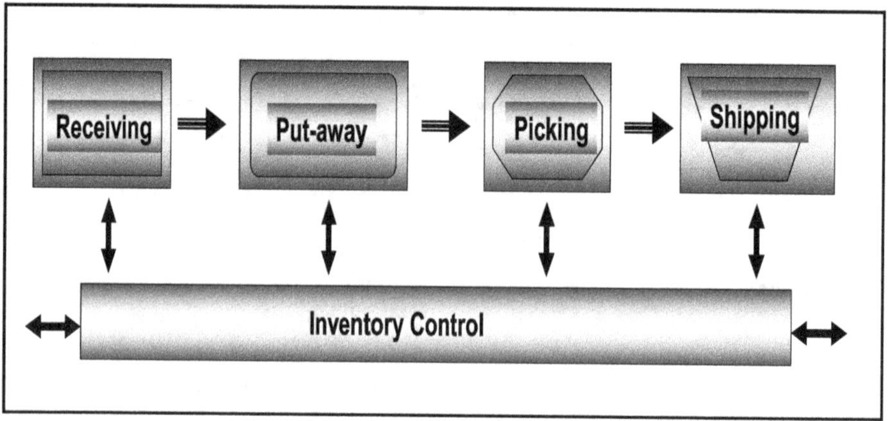

Fig. 2.10 Features of Traditional Warehouse Activity.

The item-receiving and put-away process within warehouses can be dramatically improved through automatic or semi-automatic capture of data and the resultant immediacy of information. Thus, some basic system requirements include-

(a) Bar code reader terminals

These are usually portable but may be fixed position depending upon needs where bar code labels need to be produced in-house the system must also include appropriate printers and supporting software.

Quality of print is also very important requirement. Good quality bar code permits them to perform as effective data carriers. Poor quality while not necessarily introducing errors may be difficult or impossible to read. Fig. 2.11 shows a model bar coding illustration.

Fig. 2.11 Bar Coding Representations.

(b) *Software* to control the transfer of data from terminal to the host and make sensible use of the data obtained.

2.3.2.2 Picking and packaging

In manual picking processes, the picker can be given a picking list, downloaded in to a portable data terminal, which through an appropriate display can direct the picker to the items required by using appropriate software and scanning.

Picking may be more or less optimized. Picked items are packaged to consignments. They are labeled and identified with appropriate machine data carriers as shown in Fig. 2.12.

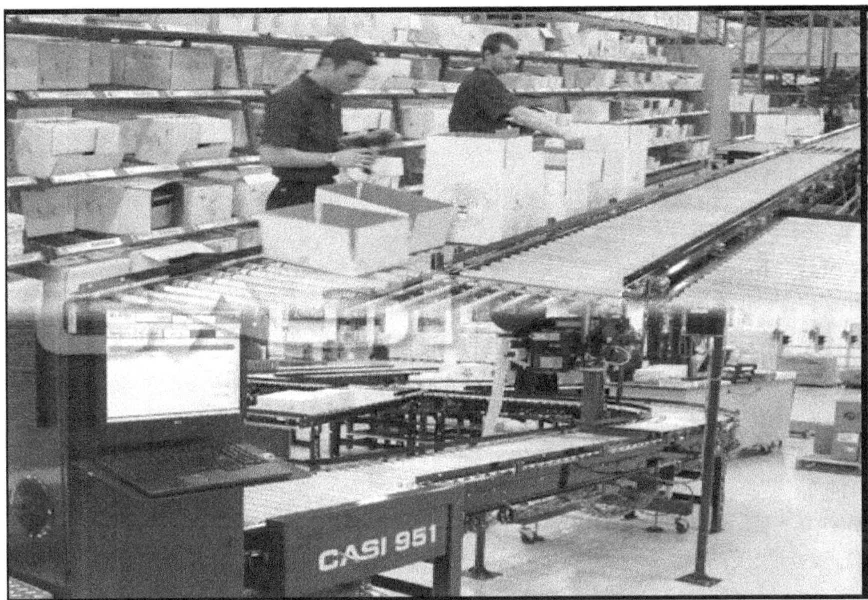

Fig. 2.12 Picture Showing the Consignments of Picked Items.

Packaging of goods is another area where suitable identification can yield benefits in better supporting the handling and shipping of items and the needs of others further down the supply chain, through to retailers.

2.3.2.3 Shipping

Getting goods out of a ware-house is an efficient and effective manner can be greatly assisted by having some form of machine readable identification.

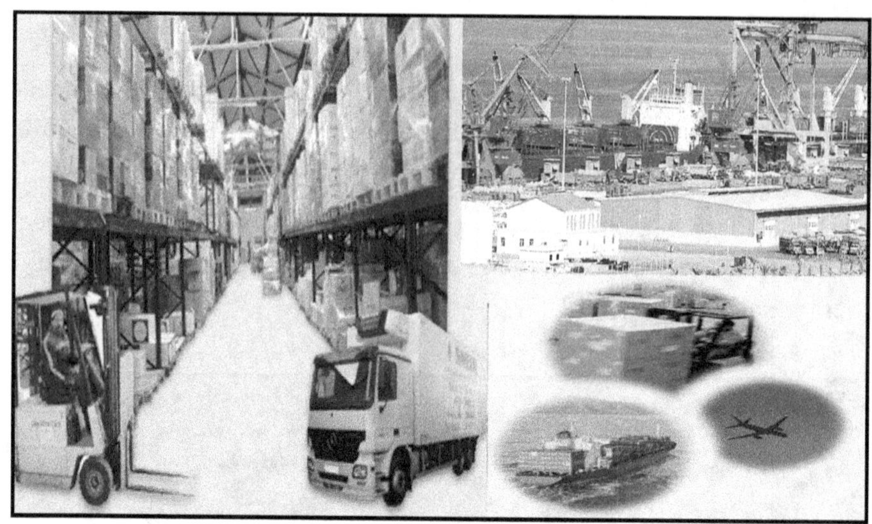

Fig. 2.13 Picture Showing the Shipping of Items.

Shipping documentation may also benefit from the use of bar coding for document tracking and in machine-readable form.

COMMUNICATION SKILLS, PHARMACEUTICAL CARE, PATIENT COUNSELING AND COMPLIANCE

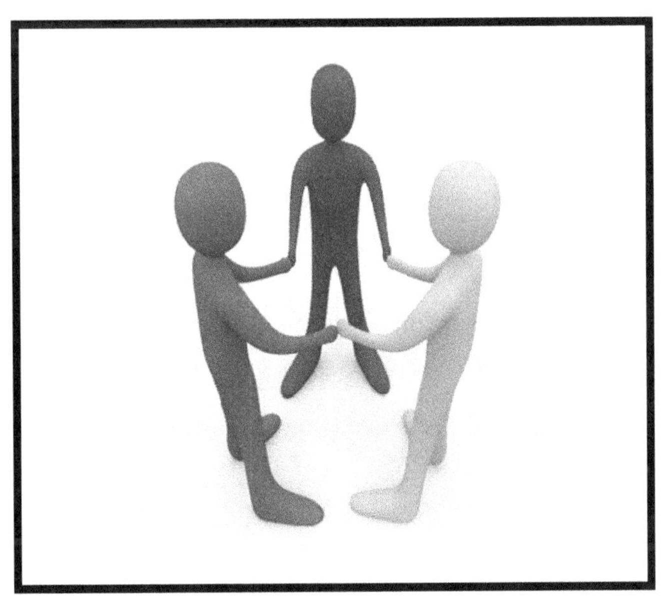

3.1 Communication Skills

"We all use language to communicate, to express ourselves, to get our ideas across, and to connect with the person to whom we are speaking. When a relationship is working, the act of communicating seems to flow relatively effortlessly. When a relationship is deteriorating, the act of communicating can be as frustrating as climbing a hill of sand."

- Chip Rose

Communication is the activity of conveying information. Communication requires a sender, a message, and an intended recipient, although the receiver need not be present or aware of the sender's intent to communicate at the time of communication; thus communication can occur across vast distances in time and space. Communication requires that the communicating parties share an area of communicative commonality. The communication process is complete once the receiver has understood the sender.

Communication is a complex process that we all use constantly, often with little thought or serious consideration. Pharmacists rely primarily on sight and hearing in professional situations and occasionally perhaps, on touch.

To be professionally effective pharmacist, pharmacists need to be aware of:

(a) The different message they are sending.

(b) How these could be perceived.

(c) The ways in which we interpret these messages, which can be inaccurate.

(d) How to ensure that communication is tailored to the situation and to the audience, and supports good pharmacy practice and human relations.

The various steps which involve patient communication are shown in following cycle:

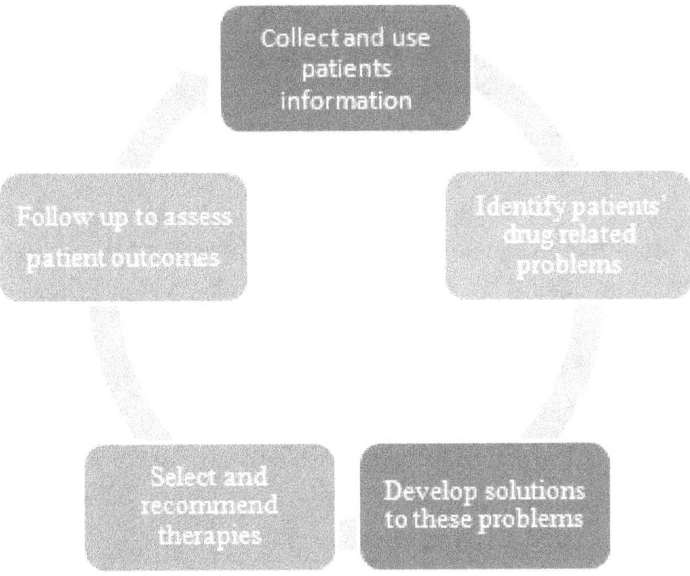

Fig. 3.1 The Pharmacy Care Process.

3.1.1 Empathy

This is an important first step in establishing communication skills. Empathy is the ability to see and feel what the world is like for another person. Every individual is unique and special, and it can take considerable effort to develop the skills to react appropriately to the uniqueness of every person we meet. By using basic communication skills of listening and observing closely, an appropriate approach can be developed which will enhance communication using the knowledge and skills.

3.1.2 Non-Verbal Communication

When we first meet someone, before a word is spoken, we form an impression of them, as they do of us. Without our knowledge, our brain and sensory organs are processing large amounts of information (What do they look like? How are they dressed? How old they are? Are they hostile or shy? Do I like what I see or smell?).

The first impression can have a significant influence on how we react to others. Further contact with someone will add and support our first impression or we may be required to change our impression of that person.

Non-verbal communication includes messages conveyed through body posture. Non-verbal signals such as looking away, fidgeting, doing something else at the same time or allowing people to interrupt you, can also signal inattention and inhibit communication. Facial expression is an important indicator of emotional state. We instinctively observe the face to interpret another person's reaction to us.

Another form of non-verbal message is to convey information through the use of diagrams. These could be used in place of medicines labels for the illiterate or may demonstrate how to administer a dosage form such as eye drops.

3.1.3 Verbal Communication

Verbal communication takes place using the meaning of words. It can be spoken or written. The meanings of words can, however be altered by the non-verbal aspects of voice tone or emphasis.

3.1.3.1 Language

For reliable communication, it is important to use a language in which both the parties are fluent and comfortable. Medicine and pharmacy have a shared professional language and one that uses Greek and Latin terminology, which is very different from ordinary and simple language. It is most important that the appropriate form of language is used for particular person you are talking with.

3.1.3.2 Interactive communication

Two activities are principally involved in communication: the sending and receiving of messages. Effective communication and learning are essentially two-way interactive process. Both the parties are actively participating in speaking and listening and interpreting the meaning of what is happening based on their personal experience.

3.1.3.3 Listening skills

Developing good listening skills is important to promote a good interactive communication and to obtain information. It is important that the listener maintains undivided attention and is not distracted by external or internal matters.

3.1.4 Communication with the Patients

3.1.4.1 Medication history interviews

When health professionals are making decisions about the treatment, it is importance that a complete medication history is available. A well prepared, structured approach helps to avoid omissions. The following information is commonly recorded:

  (i)   Currently or recently prescribed medicines.

  (ii) Medicines purchased without prescription (OTC).

  (iii) Vaccinations.

  (iv) Alternative or traditional remedies.

  (v)   Description of reactions and allergies to medicines.

  (vi) Medicines found to be ineffective.

3.1.4.2 Labeling medicines

All containers of medicines should be clearly labeled to identify:

  (i)   The medicine.

  (ii) Dosage form, number of dosage units supplied, strength.

  (iii) Number of dose units to be taken at one time.

  (iv) Frequency and any specific precautions.

  (v)   The patient's name.

  (vi) Date of dispensing.

  (vii) Batch numbers and expiry dates for non-prescription medicines and medicines not likely to be used immediately.

3.1.4.3 Patient information leaflets (PILs)

Patient information leaflets are used to outline key information to assist patient and their caregivers for the effective and safe use of a medicine. The following information is commonly included in the PILs:

  (i)   Trade and generic name.

  (ii) Indication for which the medicine is being taken.

(iii) Administration advice.

(iv) Information on the action required if a dose is missed.

 (v) The common or serious side-effects.

(vi) Action to be taken if a side-effect is experienced.

(vii) Storage information.

(viii) Name and contact details of the institution providing information.

 (ix) Author and date of publication.

3.1.4.4 Patient medication sheets

When patients are taking several medicines, handwritten or computer-generated medication records can improve compliance and understanding. A tabular form will present the information clearly.

3.1.4.5 Medication counseling for patients

Effective patient counseling can assist patients in using their medicines safely and reliably. All the principles of effective verbal communication are important to the success of an encounter. The medication record can be used to focus an interview, supported by patient information leaflets or product demonstrations.

3.1.5 Strategies to Overcome Communication Barriers

"A barrier to communication is something that keeps meanings from meeting. Meaning barriers exist between all people, making communication much more difficult than most people seem to realize. It is false to assume that if one can talk he can communicate. Because so much of our education misleads people into thinking that communication is easier than it is, they become discouraged and give up when they run into difficulty. Because they do not understand the nature of the problem, they do not know what to do. The wonder is not that communicating is as difficult as it is, but that it occurs as much as it does."

- Reuel Howe

As a health care providers or pharmacist, it is our responsibility to assess patients and communicate with them in ways they can understand. Communication barrier includes various aspects such as patients who have difficulty in reading, older adult patients, patients with visual impairments, hearing-impaired patients, patients who speak little or no English and patients from other cultures.

According to *AORN Journal*, August 2001, by Mary E. Barich, *"If you can do only five things, the communication barrier can be overcome."* The five goals are as follows:

(a)   Creating a positive environment.

(b)   Limiting your teaching objectives.

(c)   Communicating clearly and simply.

(d)   Using multiple methods to convey your message.

(e)   Verifying understanding.

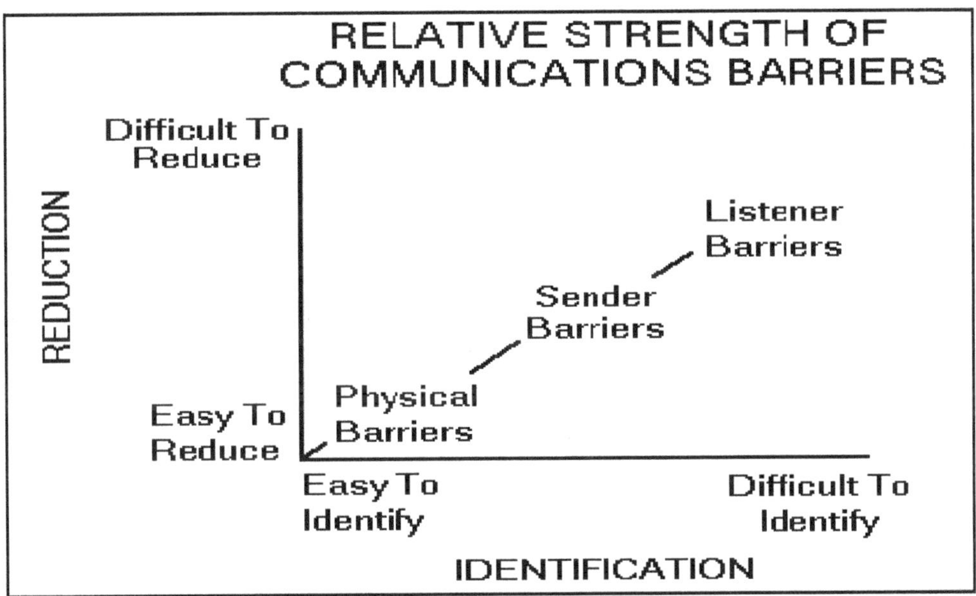

Fig. 3.2 Various Types of Barriers in Communication.

3.1.6 Patient Counseling

Counseling has become a basic component of every health care service. Counseling skills are applicable in common daily health care situations to meet specific needs of patients.

Counseling can be defined as means by which one person helps another to make a decision about an issue and act on that decision. As this communication plays a vital part in the health sector, the counselor needs to be skilled in analyzing and evaluating the human behavior. They need to know about human behavior and development, relationships, different techniques, social and cultural issues. The patient will always look for empathy, respect and sensitivity from the counselor. They would like to freely express their real concerns. They expect the counselor to give careful attention to their concern and maintain confidentiality. So it is necessary for a counselor to develop good personal qualities and communication skills to help the patient to make an informed decision. Patient counseling refers to the process of providing information, advice and assistance to help patients use their medications appropriately.

Communication is very essential in counselling. The counselor should remember that everything they do creates an impression. Thus they should be aware of their posture, facial expressions, eye contact, hand gestures, dress etc. Between 60-80 % of our message is communicated through our body language and only 7-10 % is attributable to the actual words of a conversation.

The information and advice given by the pharmacist directly to the patient or patient's representative, and may also include information about the patient's illness or recommended lifestyle changes. The information is usually given verbally, but may be supplemented with written materials. During counseling the pharmacist should assess the patient's understanding about his or her illness and its treatment and provide individualized advice and information which will assist the patient to their medications in the most safe and effective manner.

Effective patient counseling aims to produce the following results:

(a) Better patient understanding of their illness and role of medication in its treatment.

(b) Improved medication adherence.

(c) More effective drug treatment.

(d) Reduced incidence of adverse effects and unnecessary health-care cost.

(e) Improved quality of life for the patient.

(f) Better coping strategies to deal with medication related adverse effects improve professional rapport between the patient and the pharmacist.

3.1.6.1 Tips for good counseling

➤ Be relaxed and attentive. Always lean forward while talking to the patients that show our interest towards them.

➤ Keep your facial expressions relaxed and friendly.

➤ When standing, maintain a balance to our stance.

➤ Move purposefully; it shows confidence.

➤ Use your hands above the waist. Use both hands and make large gestures. Keeping the palms up is a positive gesture.

➤ Smile when appropriate; look pleasant and genuine, this shows the warmth and openness of the counselor.

➤ Always turn the face towards the patient nodding head vertically.

Avoid . . .

➤ Gestures like crossing the legs, swinging foot and tapping fingers reveals that the counselor is impatient and not interested.

➤ Avoid shifting eyes and head quickly during conversation when the patient asks a question.

➤ Avoid hair twirling, this shows that the counselor is incompetent and uncertain.

➤ Don't place the hands in front of the mouth or rub the arm or leg, this shows that the counselor is in anxiety.

➤ Avoid talking too loud or too low. When talking to the patient do not look down or frown the face, this shows that the counselor is defensive and untrustworthy.

➤ Avoid cleaning glasses, biting nails, rubbing eyes and noses.

➤ Do not look down or to the side. Look directly at the person with a sense of confidence but not overbearing or threatening in nature.

3.1.7 Communication Skills for Effective Counseling

The counseling process uses verbal and non-verbal communication skills. Verbal communication skills include language and paralinguistic features such as tone, volume, pitch and rate of speech.

(a) **Language:** When speaking to the patients use simple language and avoid using unnecessary medical words. If possible, speak the patient's own language.

(b) **Tone:** During counseling, the tone of one's voice is important. Changes in the level and range of pitch convey information about the feelings and attitude of the person speaking. The tone of the voice should be caring and reassuring.

(c) **Volume:** Ideally counseling should be conducted in a quiet private setting where it is unnecessary to raise one's voice.

(d) **Speed:** The clarity of our communication depends on our rate of speech. For good verbal communication, the pharmacist should present clear, relevant messages in a logical sequence, and at a speed which gives the patient time to think about what is being said. This will help the patient to understand and remember the concepts more easily.

(e) **Proximity:** This refers to the distance that people maintain between themselves during the counseling process.

(f) **Eye contact:** The duration of time that people look at one another during a conversation varies depending on whether they are speaking or listening. Listeners look at the speaker more often and for longer periods of time.

(g) **Facial Expression:** These can be used during counseling to demonstrate empathy towards patient. Head movements such as nodding, hand gestures and body postures also can be used to advantage.

3.1.8 Steps During Patient Counseling

Counseling is a two-way communication process and interaction between the patient and the pharmacist is essential for counseling to be effective.

3.1.8.1 Preparing for the session

The success of counseling depends upon the knowledge and skills of the counselor. The pharmacist should know as much as possible about the patient and his/her treatment details.

Another issue worth considering is the mental and physical state of patient. If a patient is in hurry, in pain or in non-communicative state, it is very difficult to counsel the patient effectively. In such situations, the aim of counseling may need to be modified, or with the patients agreement the session may be postponed to a later date.

3.1.8.2 Opening the session

The first phase of the counseling is used for information gathering. The pharmacist should introduce himself or herself to the patient and greet them by name. The pharmacist should identify the purpose of the session very clearly.

Next, the pharmacists gather information from the patient about understanding of their disease, drug treatment and use of alternative medications such as ayurvedic medication or home remedies. Using open-ended questions is a useful technique for gaining the confidence of the patient and answers all the pharmacist's questions to assess the patient's information need.

3.1.8.3 Counseling content

The counseling content is considered to be the heart of the counseling session. During this step, the pharmacist explains to the patient about his or her medications and treatment regimen. Topics commonly covered include:

- Name and strength of the medication.
- Reasons why it has been prescribed (if known), or how it works.
- How to take the medication? (how much and how often).
- Expected duration of treatment.
- Expected benefits of treatment.
- Possible adverse effects.
- Possible medications and dietary interactions.
- Advice on correct storage.
- Minimum time duration required to show therapeutic benefit.
- What to do if a dose is missed?
- Special monitoring requirements. e.g. Blood tests etc.
- Arrangement for obtaining further supplies.

3.1.8.4 Closing the session

Before closing the session, it is essential to check the patients understanding. This can be assessed by feedback questioning such as "Can you remember what this medication is for?" or "How long should you take this medication?" During discussion some of the patients information needs may have been cleared, but the patients may have new questions and doubts. It is therefore advisable to finish the session by asking the patient-"Do you have any question?" Before final closure and if time permits, summarize the main points in a logical order.

Conclusion

The pharmacist must make a reasonable effect to collect record and maintain the following information about patient receiving medical benefits:

1. Patient's name, address, telephone number, date of birth (or age) and gender.

2. Patient's individual history when important, including disease(s) state, known allergies and drug interactions.

3. A comprehensive list of medications and relevant devices.

4. Pharmacist's comment relevant to the individual's drug therapy.

3.1.9 Outcomes of Patient Counseling

With the emphasis of pharmaceutical care there are six desired outcomes of patient counseling. The patient will

1. Recognize why a prescribed medication is helpful for marinating or promoting well-being.

2. Accept the support from the health care professional in establishing a working relationship and foundation for continual interaction and consultation.

3. Develop the ability to make more appropriate medication related decisions concerning compliance or adherence.

4. Improve coping strategies to deal with medication side effects and drug interactions.

5. Become a more informed, efficient, active participant in disease treatment and self-care management.

6. Show motivation toward taking medications to improve his health states.

3.1.10 Techniques for Patient Counseling

3.1.10.1 Patient-information leaflets

Patient information leaflets are alternative forms of patient information which are used to supplement patient counseling. It includes appropriate elements as those of patient counseling which are as follows:

(i)   The name and the description of the drug.

(ii)   The dosage form, dose, route of administration and duration of drug therapy.

(iii)   Intended use of the drug and its expected action.

(iv)   Special directions and precautions for preparation, administration and use by the patient.

(v)   Common severe side or adverse effects or interactions and therapeutic contraindications that may be encountered, including their avoidance and the action required if they occurs.

(vi)   Techniques for self monitoring drug therapy.

(vii)   Proper storage.

(viii) Prescription refill information.

(ix)   Action to be taken in the event of a missed dose.

(x)   Comments relevant to the individual's drug therapy, including any other information peculiar to the specific patient or drug.

3.1.10.2 Advisory labels

The patients require adequate information so that they will take their medicine safely and effectively. The following wordings may be given on the label:

3.1.10.2.1 *For external use only*: This label must be applied to all semisolid and solid medicinal products meant for external use such as, ointments, creams, pastes and dusting powder.

3.1.10.2.2 *Not to be taken*: This label may be used on preparations that are neither administered by mouth nor used on the skin.

3.1.10.2.3 *Drowsiness warning:* Patients should be warned if their medicine is likely to cause drowsiness, dizziness and blurred vision or may impair their ability to drive or operate machine safely.

The following wordings may be written on the label:

> **Warning:** May cause drowsiness. If affected do not drive or operate machinery, avoid alcoholic drink.

3.1.10.2.4 *Potential interactions with food or drink*: The following types of wordings may be written on the label, under different conditions:

(i)   Drugs in which absorption is improved if taken before food.

> **Warning:** To be taken an hour before food or an empty stomach.

(ii)   Drugs which cause gastro-intestinal irritation or are better absorbed with food.

> **Warning:** To be taken with or after food.

(iii) Drugs such as antibiotics where the absorption is significantly decreased by the presence of food and acid in the stomach.

> **Warning:** To be taken an hour before food or an empty stomach.

(iv) Alcohol may provoke a reaction such as flushing, when taken in combination with drugs such as metronidazole.

> **Warning:** Avoid alcoholic drink.

3.1.10.2.5 *Potential interactions with medicines*: The following types of wording may be written on the label under different conditions:

(a) Drugs which chelate with calcium, magnesium and iron and are not well absorbed in the presence of these ions.

> **Warning:** Do not take milk, iron preparation with this medicine.

(b)   Drugs whose activity is reduced by aspirin.

> **Warning:** Do not take aspirin while taking the medicine.

3.1.10.2.6 *Special methods of administration*: The following wordings may be written on the label if there is some special method of administration.

(a)   The drug formulation which is required to be dissolved in the mouth.

> **Warning:** To be sucked or chewed.

(b)   The drugs which are to be absorbed through sublingual mucosa.

> **Warning:** To be dissolved under the tongue.

(c)   The drugs which are soluble in water or for powders and granules to be dispersed in water before taking.

> **Warning:** Dissolve or mix with water before taking.

(d)   The drugs which are to be used for enteric coated sustained release or having unpleasant taste.

> **Warning:** To be swallowed whole, not to be chewed.

3.1.10.2.7 *Caution in use*: The following wordings may be written on the label in order to caution a patient about certain unusual happening after taking the medicine.

(a)   The preparation which may induce photosensitization.

> **Warning:** Avoid exposure of skin to direct sunlight

(b)   The preparation which may produce unusual effect.

> **Warning:** The preparation may color the urine or stool.

(c)   The preparation which contains a high proportion of flammable solvent.

> **Warning:** Keep away from naked flame.

(d) Leaflets: These are the types of open letter or postcard designed to be handed out to the people, inserted in local newspapers for distribution, left in venues, shops and at places where they will catch a person's eye.

Leaflets are normally used to deliver useful and reusable information. The size and shape of the leaflet is a major factor in success. A leaflet that people cannot fit easily into a pocket or a bag will be thrown away. While designing a leaflet, you are expressing yourself not only with words but also with pictures and graphics. There are four clear tasks in the design of a leaflet:

1. *Decide what you want to say:* It should be clear and persuasive. If the leaflet is being produced by a group, it must discuss the overall concept together.

2. *Text editing:* The text must be persuasive, interesting to read, catchy and memorable. Always use short paragraphs and mark them with headings. Use-bullet pointed lists which are easy to read. Important things must be highlighted in different font size and colour to make a strong point.

3. *Picture design:* The pictures help to get the message across and to understand the concept clearly and thoroughly.

4. *Layout design:* The layout needs to be thought out very carefully. Work out with the rest of the group what text and pictures you will have. Using a piece of plain paper sketch out: Where the blocks of text, headings and pictures will go. The color of the text and the background also plays a vital role.

3.2 COMPLIANCE

3.2.1 Definition

In medicine, compliance describes the degree to which a patient correctly follows medical advice. Most commonly, it refers to medication or drug compliance, but may also mean use of medical appliances such as compression stockings, chronic wound care, self-directed physiotherapy exercises, or attending counseling or other courses of therapy. Both the patient and the health-care provider affect compliance, and a positive physician-patient relationship is the most important factor in improving compliance, although the high cost of prescription medication also plays a major role. Compliance is also called as adherence, concordance, or capacitance.

A WHO study estimates that only 50 % of patients suffering from chronic diseases in developed countries follow treatment recommendations. This may affect patient health, and affect the wider society when it causes complications from chronic diseases, formation of resistant infections, or untreated psychiatric illness. Compliance rates during closely monitored studies are usually far higher than in later real-world situations.

3.2.2 Factors Affecting Patient Compliance

Patient compliance can be defined as the extent to which an individual's behavior coincides with medical or health advice.

The various factors affecting patients compliance includes:

3.2.2.1 Patients

Patients who live alone are less likely to comply than those who live with another family member who can take an interest in and/or supervise their therapy. The increasing problem of drug abuse and addiction have increased the awareness and concern about becoming dependent on agents that are prescribed for legitimate medical reasons.

3.2.2.2 Disease

In patients with psychiatric disorders, the ability to corporate as well as the attitude towards the treatment may be accomplished by the illness and these individuals may be more likely than other patients to be non-compliant.

3.2.2.3 Taste of medication

Compliance problems related to the taste of the medication are not limited to children. Objections to the taste of liquid potassium chloride preparations often are raised, a number of patients discontinue taking the medication for this reason.

3.2.2.4 Administration of medication

Although patients may fully intend to comply with instructions, they may inadvertently receive the wrong quality of medication because of incorrect measurement of medication, use of inappropriate measuring devices, or incorrect use of medication administration devices.

3.2.2.5 Cost of medication

Non-compliance often occurs with the use of drugs that have relatively low cost, however it might be anticipated that patients may be even more reluctant to use the entire prescribed quantity of more expensive agents.

3.2.2.6 Patients may be asymptomatic or symptoms subside

It is understandably difficult to conceive a patient of the value of drug therapy when the patient has experienced symptoms prior to initiation of therapy.

3.2.2.7 Adverse events

The development of unpleasant effects of a drug is a likely deterrent to compliance. The adverse events (for example nausea, vomiting and hair loss) associated with the use of many antineoplastic drugs are sufficiently distressing to a number of patients that they do not take their medications in the manner intended.

3.2.2.8 Duration therapy

The rate of non-compliance becomes greater when the treatment period is long. As noted a greater risk of non-compliance should be anticipated in patients with chronic disorders, especially if discontinuation of therapy is not likely to be associated with prompt recurrence of symptoms or worsening of the illness.

3.2.2.9 Patient/health professional interaction

One of the patients need is psychological support provided in a compassionate manner, and it has been observed that patients are more inclined to comply with the instructions of a physician they know well and respect and from whom they receive information and assurance about their illness and medication.

3.2.2.10 Failure to comprehend the importance of therapy

A major for non-compliance is that the importance of the drug therapy and the potential consequences if the medication is not used according to the instructions has not been impressed upon the patient.

3.2.2.11 Poor understanding of the instructions

Prescriptions which state that the medication should be taken as directed can be the source of misunderstanding as well as serious consequences.

3.2.3 Role of Pharmacist in Improving Patient Compliance

Pharmacists have a particularly valuable opportunity to encourage compliance since their advice accompanies the actual dispensing of the medication, and they usually are the last health professional to see the patient prior to the time the medication is to be used.

3.2.3.1 Identification of the risk factors

A first step in efforts to improve compliance should be to recognize individuals who are most likely to be non-compliant as judged by a consideration of the risk factors. These factors should be taken in account in planning the patients therapy so that the simplest regimen that is, to the extent possible, compatible with the patients normal activities can be developed.

3.2.3.2 Development of treatment plan

The more complex the treatment regimen, the greater is the risk of non-compliance. So the treatment plan should be individualized on the basis of the patients need and when possible, the patient should be a participant in decisions regarding the therapeutic regimen.

3.2.3.3 Patient education

Education is the best way to improve compliance. It should be decided what information should be provided to patients about their illness and drug therapy with a patient; a distinction should be made between information and education. Patients may receive information but not understand it and use it correctly, whereas education implies understanding and behavioral changes.

(a) *Oral communication/counseling*: Oral communication is the most important component of patient education because it directly involves both the patient and the pharmacist in a two-way exchange and provides the opportunity for the patient to raise questions. For such, communication to be more effective it should be conducted in a setting that provides privacy and is free of distractions.

(b) *Written communication*: Although at the time of the visit to the physician or the pharmacist patients may understand how the medication is to be used. Later, they may not remember the details relating to the administration of the drug. Therefore, specific instructions for use should be placed on the prescription label.

3.2.3.4 Patient motivation

Many health care professional assume that patients who are knowledgeable about their illness and therapeutic regimen are likely to be more compliant. Although this premise is valid for many patients, increased patient knowledge does not necessarily alter patient behavior and compliance. Therefore there must be an awareness of the need to motivate patients to use the knowledge they have acquired to achieve optimum benefit from their therapy.

3.2.3.5 Compliance aids

(a) *Labeling*: Auxiliary labels that provide additional information regarding the use, and/or storage of the medication also will contribute to the attainment of the compliance.

(b) *Medications calendars and drug reminder charts*: Various forms, such as medication calendars have been designed and developed to assist the patient in self-administering drugs.

(c) *Special medication containers, caps and systems*: Several types of medication containers have been developed to help patients in organizing their medications and to monitor self-administration of the drugs. An example is the 28-compartment MED/SET containers. This device contains four compartments for different time prior to\for each day of the week.

(d) *Compliance packaging*: The member in which medication is packaged also has an influence on the patient compliance. For example, Blister packaging using one unit and is designed to serve as a patient-education tool for health professionals and to make it easier for patients to understand and remember to take their medications correctly at home.

(e) *Dosage forms*: For example, the development of longer acting, controlled release dosage form of calcium channel blocking agents has permitted less frequent administration of these agents, which facilitates compliance.

3.2.3.6 Monitoring therapy

(a) *Self- monitoring*: Patients should be apprised of the importance of monitoring their own treatment regimen and the response parameters.

(b) *Pharmacist monitoring*: The pharmacist is in an excellent position to detect non-compliance pertaining to drug used by being alert to situations in which the frequency of required refills is not consistent with the directions for use.

3.3   PATIENT CARE

In years past, the responsibility of the pharmacist was to dispense prescriptions accurately, provide medication counseling and answer questions of concern to the patients. Recently, however, the profession of pharmacy has adopted pharmaceutical care as its mission and thereby extended the responsibility of the pharmacist. Pharmaceutical care focuses pharmacist's attitude, behavior, commitment, concern, ethics, functions, knowledge, responsibilities and skills on the provision of drug therapy to individual patients. The goal is to achieve optimal outcomes that improve the patient quality of life. The outcomes may include:

- Cure of the disease.
- Elimination or reduction of the symptoms.
- Arresting or slowing the disease process.
- Prevention of disease.
- Diagnosis of disease.
- Desired alterations in the physiological processes.

In response to our societal needs for medication management, community pharmacists are beginning to assume the additional responsibility of increasing the effectiveness of drug therapy through the provision of pharmaceutical care. They are shifting from a dispensing focus, which emphasizes the drug product, to a patient-oriented focus, which emphasizes proper use of drug therapy for the patient.

3.3.1 Definition and Principles of Pharmaceutical Care

Pharmaceutical care as the responsible provision of drug therapy and other patient care services for the purpose of achieving outcomes related to the prevention or cure of the disease, the elimination or reduction of patients symptoms or the prevention, arrest or slowing of a disease process. It involves the process through which pharmacist in co-operation with the patient and other health-care professional design, implement and a monitor, a therapeutic plan that will produce specific therapeutic outcomes for the patient and improves patient's quality of life.

The community pharmacists are engaging in pharmaceutical care activities include

1. Nutritive services.
2. Blood pressure monitoring.

3. Diabetes training.

4. Health screenings.

5. Asthma training.

6. Patient education programs.

7. Immunizations.

8. AIDS specialty services.

9. Anti-coagulation services.

Furthermore, contemporary pharmacy practitioners are discovering that providing comprehensive patient care is more satisfying than only dispensing medications. Thus, while the prescription and non-prescription drug products are still the prominent domain of the community pharmacy, the patient-centered approach is diffusing throughout community practice settings and advancing the profession.

Pharmacist providers of pharmaceutical care engage in a series of sequential steps to ensure that individual patient receive cost-effective pharmacotherapy that results in optional therapeutic outcomes. These steps include having the pharmacist.

(a) Establish a committed relationship with individual patients.

(b) Collect, synthesize and interpret relevant patient information.

(c) Define and prioritize the potential and actual medication related problems of the patients.

(d) Establish a desired pharmacotherapeutic outcome for each medication related problem.

(e) Determine feasible pharmacotherapeutic alternatives to achieve each desired outcomes.

(f) Select the best pharmacotherapeutic solution based upon individual patient circumstances.

(g) Design a monitoring plan to determine if the desired pharmacotherapeutic outcome has been achieved.

(h) Implement the individualized pharmacotherapeutic and monitoring plans and evaluate and document the results of pharmacotherapeutic and monitoring plans.

OTC MEDICATIONS AND HEALTH SCREENING SERVICES

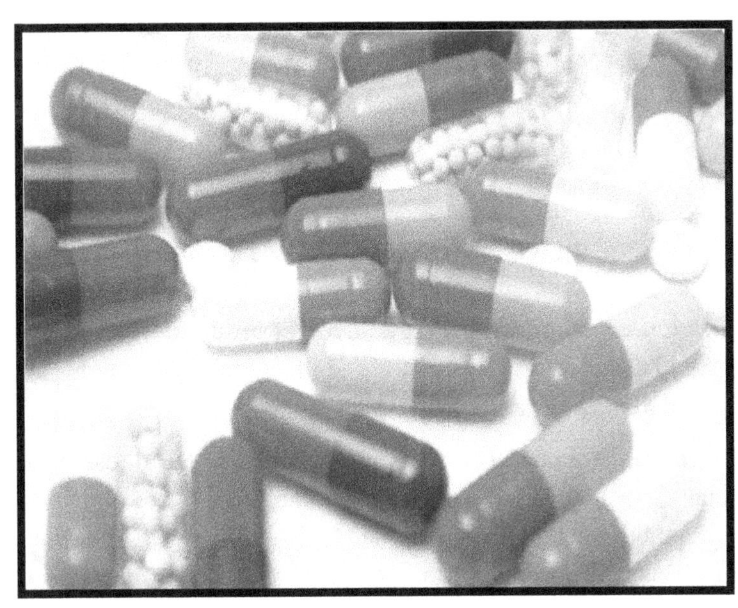

4.1 OTC MEDICATIONS

In past one decade, people are becoming increasingly interested in "self-care". This means they are more getting involved decisions about health care of their family and themselves. One reason for this is availability of variety of alternative and complimentary approaches towards medicine.

Now people are involving in ingestion of number of non-traditional agents and extra nutritional supplements like vitamins, herbs, minerals, nutraceuticals etc. As per general surveys carried out – use of medicines that can be obtained without consulting a physician are also increased.

Medications can be broadly classified into two categories:

1. Prescription controlled and
2. Prescription de-controlled drug.

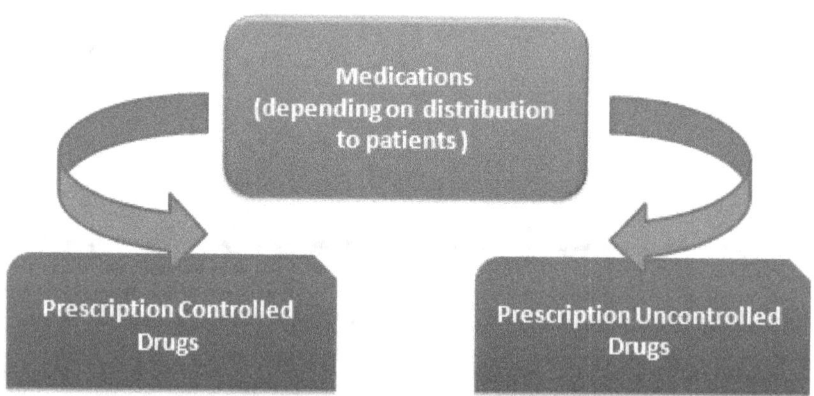

Fig. 4.1 Various Categories of Medications.

Prescription controlled*:* This class involves all the drugs and medicines which need a signed prescription of eligible authority i.e. a physician or a Registered Medical Practitioner (RMP).

Prescription de-controlled: This class includes all those drugs and medicines which do not require a written prescription of a physician or a medical practitioner. Such medicines can be directly purchase over the chemist bench. Those drugs are therefore called as over the Counter (OTC) drugs or Non Prescribed Drugs (NPDs).

4.1.1 OTC Medications: General Introduction

OTC medications are those medications that can be obtained over the counter or from the chemist bench without any prescription of a RMP and consultation with a physician. It can be suggested that these have little significant pharmacological activity and therefore the physicians need not to be very much concerned about their use by the patients themselves. Hence, medicines can be categorized on the basis of their distribution to patients into prescription and NPDs.

The various studies suggest that NPDs are used primarily for symptomatic relief and not as substitutes for prescription drugs or visits to the Physician, except when access to professional care is limited and they are meant only for non-threatening symptoms.

Various factors influence use of non-prescription medication. Elderly persons and women are the most frequent users of NPDs. Patients with higher educational levels, less time available for physician visits, or fewer accesses to professional medical care are more likely to use non prescription medications. The factor which exhibits the greatest influence on use of non-prescription medication is the number of recent symptoms and frequency of visits to the physician. Use of non-prescription and prescription drugs is partially correlated because less healthy individuals use more or both types of drugs. It is not worthy that as the cost to the patient or prescription and non-prescription drugs increases fewer of each type are purchased per capita.

4.1.2 OTC Medications: History

Glancing at mid 1850's majority of health care was provided by lay practitioners, not by physicians and medicines were administered at home only. In 1860's the preparation of remedies at home was replaced by purchasing of patient medicines. By 1905 the market of the patent drugs was at its peak. However till 1920 due to intense economic and political struggle changed preference of home care to professional care, resulted in decline in public demand and use of patent medicines.

Peoples fear towards hospitals and physicians was replaced by concern about dangers of self-care. Coincidently there was a large sale of prescription drugs. The market of patent drugs was overcome by OTC drugs which were mainly for symptomatic effect.

Today, people rely on physicians and hospitals but the trend of self-care is at its peak and therefore OTC medications have their own significance.

4.1.3 OTC Medications: Reasons for Prevailing

There are number of reasons due to which OTC medications are highly popular among common people. Some of the reasons include:

4.1.3.1 Shortage of time and comfort

Usually people in cities and towns, due to their hectic routines, do not get proper time for visiting physician and for getting proper medications. But OTC medications are very less time consuming and easily available.

4.1.3.2 Cheaper in price

In country like India, where more than 55 % of the total population is just near the poverty line, people majority are weak to visit physicians for small health problems and hence prefer for non-prescribed drugs which are comparatively cheaper.

4.1.3.3 Availability

Most of the NPDs are very easily available and at all places. Due to their good availability, they are easily preferred by common people for daily health problems.

4.1.3.4 Level of literacy and awareness

Many of people have either very low level of awareness due to which they do not prefer to visit a physician. Even such people on counseling a chemist may opt for NPDs.

4.1.3.5 Self-care

Now a day people with high literacy and awareness prefer the use of OTC medications. This is because of increase of self-care in people that they can take care of their own health.

4.1.3.6 Advertisements

Most of the OTC medications producing industry gives attractive advertisement for increasing the purchase of the medication. Also people due to previous experiences or due to the experiences of other people normally opt for OTC medications.

4.1.4 OTC Medications: Significance

(i) OTC medications are comparatively cheaper and because of poverty prevailing in India, people favor NPDs.

(ii) An increased trend for self-care and increased tendency of patients to maintain their own health, force them to pay more attention towards NPDs.

(iii) The chemist himself may prescribe NPDs. This practice is commonly seen in India.

(iv) NPDs are considered as time saving medications. Some patient's do not want to spend much time at physician's clinic.

(v) NPDs have generally lesser number of side effects as compared to prescription medications.

4.1.4.1 Benefits and risks of switching from prescription drugs to OTC medications

Possible benefits

1. Increased access.
2. Decreased frequency of visits to physicians, leading to lower healthcare costs.
3. Improved education of consumers.
4. Increased autonomy of patients.
5. Decreased cost to third party players.

Possible risks

1. Inaccurate diagnosis.
2. Delay in obtaining needed therapy.
3. Use of suboptimal therapy.
4. Drug resistance.
5. Increased costs to patients due to side effects, adverse effects and drug interactions.
6. Failure to follow label instructions.
7. Perceived loss of control by physicians.

4.1.5 OTC Medications: Vulnerable Group of Users

Some people may be more likely to have side effects or other problems upon using OTC products. These groups, particularly, should take proper precautions before opting for OTC medications. Such groups include the following-

- Children.
- Women who are trying to get pregnant/ are pregnant or are breast-feeding.
- Geriatric Patients.
- Special Groups: People having health problems & people taking prescription drugs.

4.1.5.1 Do's and don'ts for each class

4.1.5.1.1 *Children*

- Pay close attention to the dose information on the drug label. Make sure you give the right amount of medicine to your child at the right times.
- Labels for liquid medicines show measurements in both teaspoons (tsp) and milliliters (mL). Keep in mind that 1 tsp is not the same as 1 mL which actually represents 5 mL.
- A kitchen teaspoon may not hold the right amount of liquid medicine. Always use the measuring device that comes with the OTC medicine. Measuring devices include droppers, spoons made just for measuring liquid medicine, and cups that are labeled with both tsp and mL. Your pharmacist can also give you a proper measuring device. If you need help using the device, ask your pharmacist to explain you how to use the device.
- Measure carefully. If you're giving liquid medicine that requires using a measuring cup, set the cup on a level surface. Then pour the medicine into it.

Concept of child resistant packaging

Child-resistant caps are designed for repeated use to make it difficult for children to open. It's best to store all medicines including vitamins and supplements where children can neither see nor reach them. Containers of pills should not be left on the kitchen counter as a reminder. Purses and briefcases are among the worst places to hide drugs from curious kids. Since the children are natural mimics, it's a good idea not to take medicine in front of them. They may be tempted to "play house" with your medicine later on. Be especially careful with iron-containing supplements. Iron is the leading cause of accidental fatal poisonings in children below age of three.

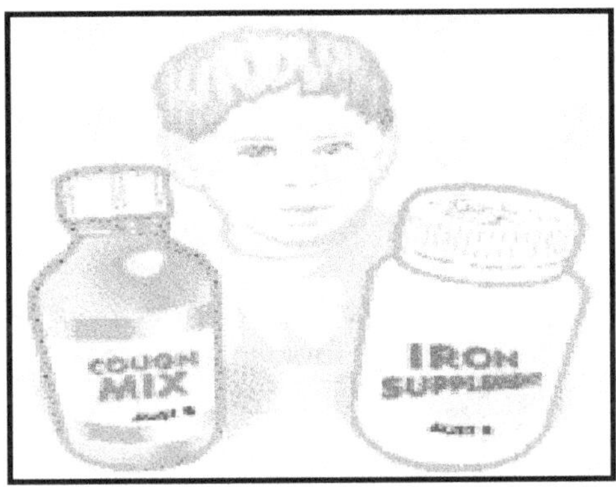

4.1.5.1.2 *Pregnancy*

The following are some basic guidelines for taking medicine when you're pregnant:

- Always talk to your doctor before taking any medicine or herbal health product when you're pregnant.
- If possible, avoid using medicines during your first trimester. This is when the risk to your baby is highest.
- Acetaminophen is usually safe for short-term pain relief during pregnancy.
- Avoid using aspirin during pregnancy. It can cause low birth weight and problems during delivery.
- Avoid using non-steroidal anti-inflammatory drugs (NSAIDs), especially during the third trimester of pregnancy. NSAIDs can cause heart problems in your baby. NSAIDs include ibuprofen, ketoprofen and naproxen.

4.1.5.1.3 *Breast-feeding women*

The following are some basic guidelines for taking medicine when you're breast-feeding.

- Talk to your doctor before taking any medicine or herbal health product when you're breast-feeding.

- Acetaminophen and NSAIDs, such as ibuprofen, usually provide safe pain relief for women who are breast-feeding.

- While breast-feeding, avoid using aspirin. Aspirin is secreted out in the breast milk. It can cause rashes and bleeding problems in nursing babies.

- Limit long-term use of antihistamines. Antihistamines is also secreted come out in the breast milk. They may cause side effects in nursing infants, such as drowsiness, crankiness, crying and sleep problems. Antihistamines may also decrease the amount of milk production. Antihistamines include brompheniramine, chlorpheniramine, dimenhydrinate, diphenhydramine and doxylamine.

- If you need to take an oral medicine, take it right after nursing or before your baby's longest sleep period.

- Watch your baby for signs of side effects. These signs can include a rash, trouble breathing, a headache or other symptoms that your baby didn't have before you took the medicine.

4.1.5.1.4 *Geriatric patients*

- If you use NSAIDs, you may be at risk of kidney disease and gastrointestinal (GI) bleeding.

- The decongestant pseudoephedrine can increase blood pressure in your eyes. This can lead to glaucoma. Pseudoephedrine also reacts badly with many other drugs, such as beta-blockers, indomethacin, methyldopa, antidepressants, insulin and some products that treat low blood sugar.

- If you take any drugs for a seizure problem, you should not use pseudoephedrine.

- If you use a monoamine oxidase inhibitor (MAOI), avoid using pseudoephedrine or the cough medicine dextromethorphan. Pseudoephedrine and dextromethorphan can change the way MAOIs work in your system. MAOIs include isocarboxazid, phenelzine, selegiline and tranylcypromine. Antihistamines can cause drowsiness and blurred vision, which may increase your risk of falling. These medicines can also cause dry mouth and trouble urinating.

Age: dose it really matter?

FDA-approved age limits are clearly marked on the labels of most nonprescription products; however, various manufacturers have begun supplying their own pediatric dosing charts. Unfortunately, medication errors are more common than we think. These medication errors can occur in hospitals, pharmacies, or even in your own home. Before purchasing non-prescription products, always examine the label closely. It is vital for you to know the minimum age for safe use. Many products have a clear age warning such as, "children under 6 years of age; consult a doctor." These age limits appear on the product label because the product may harm children below that age.

4.1.5.1.5 *Other special groups*

People with health problems may be at higher risk of having problems when taking OTC drugs. Talk to your doctor before taking an OTC medicine if you have one of the following conditions or any other health problem:

- Breathing problems, such as asthma, emphysema or bronchitis.
- Bleeding disorders.
- Diabetes.
- Enlarged prostate gland.
- Epilepsy.
- Glaucoma.
- Gout.
- Heart disease.
- High blood pressure.
- Immune system problems.
- Kidney disease.
- Liver problems.
- Parkinson's disease.
- Psychiatric problems.
- Stroke.
- Thyroid problems.

4.1.6 OTC Medications: List of Commonly Employed Medications

There are many categories of drugs that are considered OTC medications. Some of these categories are used more popular than others. NPDs involve use of major percentage of analgesics (39 %), laxatives (17 %), vitamins (5 %), anti-ulcer agents / antacids (4 %) and anti-histaminic agents / cold cough remedies (2 %).

Table 4.1 Few of Commonly Employed OTC Medications.

Analgesics and Antipyretics	
Drug Name	*Strength & Dosage Form*
Acetaminophen	325 mg tablet,160 mg/5 ml suspension
Aspirin	81 mg chewable tablet
Aspirin (Enteric Coated)	325 mg EC tablet
Ibuprofen	200 mg tablet, 100mg/5 ml suspension
Ibuprofen	100 mg easy swallow coated tablet
Antacids/GI Meds	
Bismuth Subsalicylate	262 mg,262 mg/15 ml suspension
Calcium Carbonate	500 mg chewable tablet
Famotidine	10 mg tablets
Loperamide	2 mg capsule,1 mg/5ml solution
Omeprazole	20 mg tablet
Psyllium (Fiber Therapy)	powder
Magnesium Citrate	oral solution
Simethicone	80 mg chewable tablet, 40 mg/0.6 ml suspension
Cough/Cold/Allergy	
Brompheniramine/Pseudoephedrine	elixir
Cepacol	oral lozenge
Chlorpheniramine	4 mg tablet
Diphenhydramine	25 mg capsule, 12.5 mg/5 ml syrup
Guaifenesin/Dextromethorphan	Syrup
Loratadine	10 mg tablet
Loratadine with Pseudoephedrine	10 mg/240 mg ER tablet
Oxymetazoline	0.05 % nasal spray
Pseudoephedrine	30 mg tablet, 30 mg/5 ml syrup
Pseudoephedrine 12-hour	120 mg ER tablet

Table 4.1 *Contd...*

Analgesics and Antipyretics	
Drug Name	*Strength & Dosage Form*
Vitamin and Mineral Supplements	
Calcium Carbonate	500 mg chewable tablet
Calcium Carbonate with Vitamin D	tablet
Ferrous Gluconate	324 mg tablets
Flintstones Complete MVI	Children's chewable
Multivitamin	tablet
Multivitamin with Minerals	tablet
Calcium Carbonate	500 mg chewable tablet

4.1.7 OTC Medications: Rational Drug Use

Rational drug use is conventionally defined as use of appropriate, efficacious, safe and cost effective drug given for the right indication in the right dose, formulation, right interval and right duration of time. OTC drugs serve a good purpose in places where drugs cannot be readily brought from pharmacies with prescription; the pharmacist should not prescribe if the diagnosis is uncertain or require highly potent agents.

Frequently, pharmacists sell vitamins, tonics, iron preparations and cough mixtures to the patients for the treatment they desire and not the genuine treatment they actually need. Pharmacist dispenses vitamins for some diseases like stress, menopause symptoms, anxiety etc. which are very far off from vitamin deficiency symptoms.

Rational use of OTC drugs is very important and requires the same systematic approach as for different prescribed medicines. Care must be taken to ensure that recommended OTC products are not contraindicated in a particular patient. The OTC medications should be prescribed until only it is needed. The pharmacist should provide all the important and necessary information to the patients for effective drug therapy.

4.1.8 OTC Medications: Patient Counselling and Pharmacist

The increasing trend of inclination towards over the counter status has implications for the primary health care team as well as for consumers and patients. Better information for patients could improve the safety of over the counter medicines, but better systems need to be devised for reporting adverse reactions. "*Collaborative care*" could bring pharmacists, doctors and patients to a platform where there is a need to discuss how they will respond to self-medication practices, and ways of motivating pharmacists for advising patients need to be found. Improved communication between pharmacists and doctors could bring health care professionals into a new and more constructive interaction with each other and with the patient.

4.1.9 Implications for Pharmacist

A more optimistic scenario envisages greater co-operation between doctors and pharmacists to ensure that patients get the best possible advice, both on diagnosis from doctors and on medication from pharmacists. These positive developments need to be strongly encouraged and developed. Current obstacles to greater cooperation include the separate locations of doctors and pharmacists and the regulations which tie the pharmacist to the shop during opening hours. Freeing pharmacists to participate in more joint activities in undergraduate medical teaching, vocational training for general practitioners, and continuing professional development would help both professions.

Better communication is not only vital for individual prescriptions but also for policy making in both practices and pharmacies. Practice prescribing policies should take account of pharmacy policies for recommendation of over the counter products and vice versa, so that patients receive consistent message. Mechanisms similar to those used in the development of general practice formularies should be applied to formularies of over the counter drugs, with the provision that pharmacy customers have the right to choose drugs other than those in formulary.

4.1.9.1 Family pharmacist: need of the hour

In the changing scenario and circumstances, the concept of Family Pharmacist is being adopted by the developing countries. Family pharmacist may serve as an important source of right drug information about OTC medications for pediatrics, geriatrics and breast-feeding mothers. This in-depth subject knowledge coupled with the clinical experiences may help the breast-feeding mother in searching safe and appropriate OTC medications. Even if no assistance is sought, it becomes the ethical and moral responsibility of hospital and community pharmacist to pass on the relevant facts about the various adverse and side effects associated with OTC's. The awareness among the OTC consumers may be created on mass scale through proper advertising, publicity, exhibitions, seminars and symposia etc.

The pharmacist should hold a detailed discussion with the pediatricians, physicians and drug retailers to choke out and formulate effective plans and strategies to guide the breast-feeding mothers in this regard. Breast-feeding mothers are also suggested not to hesitate in consulting an experienced pharmacist before going for OTC medications.

Pharmacist working at hospitals and those serving the community in different capacities should play a vital role as they are in intimate contact with the general public. They should serve as the guiding force to ensure the safety of OTC drug consumers as in such cases both child and the mother are at risk if due attention is not taken with regard to the safety aspects.

4.1.9.2 Appropriate patient counseling

For pharmacists the widening scope for self-medication brings different challenges. It might seem to create the possibility of greater profits through increased sales, but in the longer term it could reduce income through the loss of dispensing fees and the associated professional allowance and could even threaten the viability of some pharmacies. More importantly, however, the professional input into the patient's choice of medicine could be lost unless a mechanism can be found for rewarding professional advice rather than just the dispensing of medicines. If doctors do not rise to the challenges of greater self-medication, patients may turn to pharmacists instead. If pharmacists were to exploit this opportunity to extend their role in direct opposition to doctors the already wary relations between the two professions could deteriorate further. This is unlikely to benefit patients.

4.1.9.3 Communication: an essential tool

Better communication is also vital not just about individual prescriptions for individual patients but about policy making in both practices and pharmacies. Practice prescribing policies should take account of pharmacies' policies on the recommendation of over the counter products, and vice versa, so that patients receive consistent messages. Mechanisms similar to those used in the development of general practice formularies should be applied to formularies of over the counter drugs, with the provision that pharmacy customers have the right to choose drugs other than those in the formulary.

4.1.9.4 In-depth subject knowledge: Its proper application

In order to impart the relevant drug information to the OTC consumers, it is mandatory for a pharmacist to have sound subject knowledge. He should be well versed and familiar with the suitable drug information like dose, dosing schedule/dosing regimen, adverse and side effects, drug interactions etc. At the same time, he must be able to apply this knowledge at appropriate time for the benefit of the consumer.

Conduction of various symposia, seminars, talks and exhibitions on related matters among medico-professionals may also prove beneficial for them.

4.1.9.5 May I help you? – Inculcation of helping attitude

It is very important for a pharmacist to inculcate certain sets of qualities like patience, co-operation, helpful and compassionate attitude, in order to achieve the target of counseling of OTC consumers successfully. Dealing the consumers sympathetically and in a proper psychologically manner will leave a strong impact on them. A proper interactive session with the consumer may prove helpful in developing a fruitful association between pharmacist and consumer, which will ultimately serve the purpose.

4.1.9.6 Pharmacist-doctor-patient: A vital triangular relationship

A more optimistic scenario envisages greater co-operation between pharmacists, doctors and nurses to ensure that patients get the best possible advice, both on diagnosis from doctors and on medication from pharmacists (Fig. 3.1). Evidence that this is happening comes from the increasing number of initiatives in which doctors and pharmacists are forging links to improve patient's use of medicines. These positive developments need to be strongly encouraged and developed.

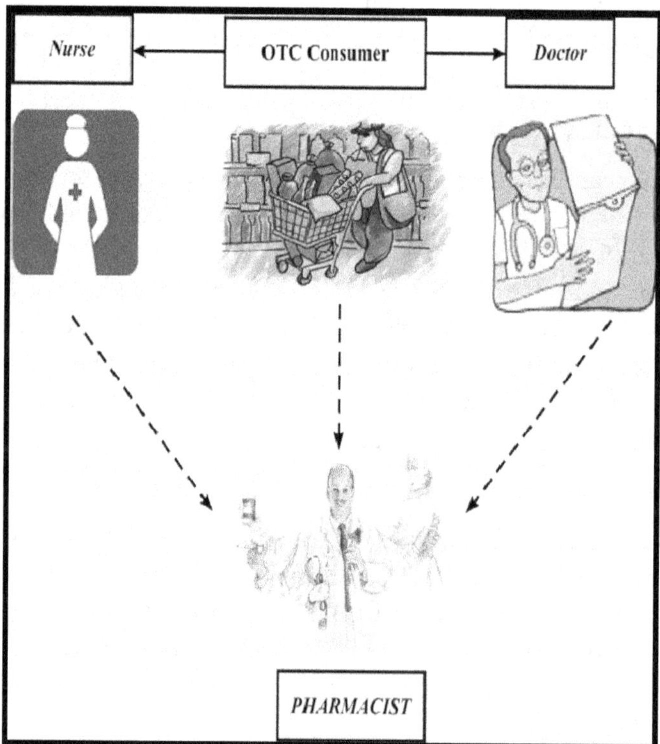

Fig. 4.2 Diagrammatic Representation depicting Triangular Relationship between Pharmacist, Doctors & Nurses and OTC Consumers.

4.1.10 Hospital and community pharmacist: essential component of triangle

A Community and Hospital Pharmacist can play a vital role in accomplishment of this job in a more comprehensive and effective manner. Pharmacist can be a major source of information to the patients residing in the rural and backward areas where a proper dialogue between the patient and a doctor is not feasible due to certain range of factors such as overpopulation, illiteracy, poverty, prevalence of superstitions and lack of medical facilities in such areas.

A community and hospital pharmacist can convey their message to the patients via various modes like verbal discussions, presentations through charts and video clippings, explanations of significant pictograms, and motivating people to increase their awareness about the employed OTC medications.

The increasing scope for self medication and its likely consequences can be seen as a shift from "*primary care*" of both minor and stable health care problems to "*self care*". Whether this transition occurs smoothly or not depends to a large extent on the attitudes and responses of the primary health care professionals involved, and whether they view this as a positive or negative development. It will also depend on how well informed and equipped the consumers are to take on the burden of self-care.

These changes could bring together the health care professionals involved (pharmacists, doctors and nurses) into a new and more constructive interaction with each other and with the patient. The need of the hour is that the pharmacist particularly Community Pharmacist should come forward to join their hands together to spread the awareness and relevant drug information among OTC consumers especially in rural and backward areas where there is utmost requirement.

One effective strategy may be the *Mass Movement* of all the Medico-Professionals like Pharmacists, Doctors and Nurses, which have the direct interactions with the OTC consumers to make the mission target oriented and successful.

4.2 HEALTH SCREENING SERVICES

4.2.1 Introduction

Screening is a public health service in which members of a defined population, who do not necessarily perceive they are at risk of, or are already affected by a disease or its complications, are asked a question or offered a test, to identify those individuals who are more likely to be helped than harmed by further tests or treatment to reduce the risk of a disease or its complications. Screening has important ethical differences from clinical practice as the health service is targeting apparently healthy people, offering to help individuals to make better informed choices about their health.

Certain tests are performed in order to diagnose disease or the extent/ stage of the disease. These tests are done at almost every health screening centres which are commonly available in community centres. These tests are called as Health Screening Tests e.g. Estimation of blood glucose, blood cholesterol, blood pressure, electrocardiograph and lung function test.

These tests may or may not prescribe by the physician. These tests do not have any side effects and thus people can themselves carry out such tests to check and monitor their health status. These tests can be performed at regular intervals of time in order to keep a check upon health and the disease.

4.2.2 Types of Health Screening Tests

Health screening tests can be categorized as-

4.2.2.1 Primary health screening tests

These tests are performed either when the physician prescribe or when a patient himself undergo such tests after the onset of the symptoms. Such test helps in diagnosing the disease and its stage. Primary health screening is also called as clinical screening or diagnostic screening.

4.2.2.2 Secondary health screening tests

These tests are performed after the diagnoses of the disease or its stage. These tests are done for mitigation of disease or to check its re-occurrence. Such tests are only carried out when the physician prescribes them.

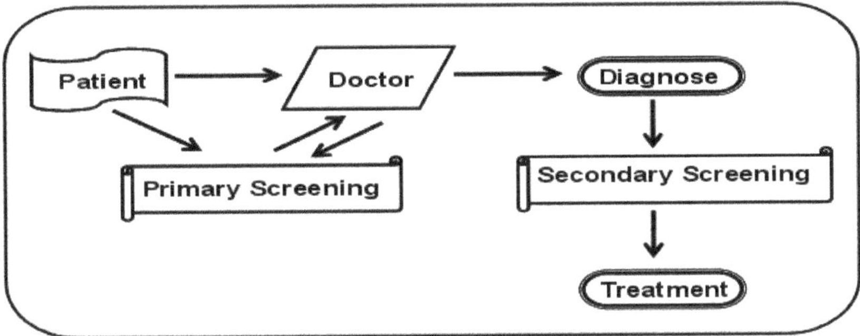

Fig. 4.3 Relationship between Primary and Secondary Screening

4.2.3 Significance of Health Screening Services

The health screening services are very important and are highly significant because of the following reasons:

(a) *Accuracy and reliability:* These are very small tests and thus accurate and can be trusted for over a perfect diagnosis of disease.

(b) *Easily available:* Primary health care tests are easily available in the nearby community or health screening centres. Even certain pharmacists can perform such tests like blood pressure, blood glucose estimation etc.

(c) *Cost effective:* These tests do not involve high cost. Such tests can be afforded by most of the population whenever they feel need of them i.e. at a point of occurrence of symptoms etc.

(d) *Can be performed anywhere:* Today most of the tests can be performed by digital portable devices and thus can be carried out anywhere. Even the costs of the digital devices are not too high and a common man can easily afford for such devices.

(e) *Side-effects:* Certain secondary health screening services have their own side effects but no side effects or adverse effects on the body were observed with primary health screening.

4.2.4 Importance of Laboratory Test Results

(i) To assess the therapeutic and adverse effects of the drugs.

(ii) To determine the proper drug dose and dosing interval (dosing regimen).

(iii) Assess the need of additional or alternate drug therapy.

4.2.5 Lung Function Test

Lung function tests (also called *pulmonary function tests or PFTs*) to evaluate how well your lungs work. The tests determine how much air your lungs can hold, how quickly you can move air in and out of your lungs, and how well your lungs put oxygen into and remove carbon dioxide from your blood. The tests can diagnose lung diseases, measure the severity of lung problems, and check to see how well treatment for a lung disease is working.

There are certain tests called as lung function test which are performed to check the capacity of lung, to check the force by which a person can inhale and exhale as well as the capacity of lungs to diffuse into the body fluids (blood). In overall, it checks how efficiently the lungs work. There are certain tests which can be performed to check the efficiency of lungs.

4.2.5.1 Spirometery

It is the oldest method of testing lung functioning and thus very important. In this test, the patient is require to breath very forcefully into the mouthpiece which is attached to an electronic recording device called as spirogram. The spirogram records the information and present the information in the form of chart and the chart called as spirograph. The various parameters which can be calculated using this test include: TLC (Total Lung Capacity), FVC (Forced Vital Capacity), FEV (Forced Expiratory Volume), FEF (Forced Expiratory Flow), PEF (Peak Expiratory Flow), ERV (Expiratory Reserve Volume), RV (Residual Volume) and IRV (Inspiratory Reserve Volume).

(i)   *Forced vital capacity (FVC):* This measures the amount of air you can exhale with force after you inhale as deeply as possible.

(ii) *Forced expiratory volume (FEV):* This measures the amount of air you can exhale with force in one breath. The amount of air you exhale may be measured at 1 second (FEV1), 2 seconds (FEV2), or 3 seconds (FEV3). FEV1 divided by FVC can also be determined.

(iii) *Forced expiratory flow 25 % to 75 %:* This measures the air flow halfway through an exhale.

(iv) *Peak expiratory flow (PEF):* This measures how quickly you can exhale. It is usually measured at the same time as your forced vital capacity (FVC).

(v)   *Maximum voluntary ventilation (MVV):* This measures the greatest amount of air you can breathe in and out during one minute.

(vi) *Slow vital capacity (SVC):* This measures the amount of air you can slowly exhale after you inhale as deeply as possible.

(vii) *Total lung capacity (TLC):* This measures the amount of air in your lungs after you inhale as deeply as possible.

(viii) *Functional residual capacity (FRC):* This measures the amount of air in your lungs at the end of a normal exhaled breath.

(ix) *Residual volume (RV):* This measures the amount of air in your lungs after you have exhaled completely. It can be done by breathing in helium or nitrogen gas and seeing how much is exhaled.

(x) *Expiratory reserve volume (ERV):* This measures the difference between the amount of air in your lungs after a normal exhale (FRC) and the amount after you exhale with force (RV).

4.2.5.2 Gas diffusion test

It is performed to check the alveolar capacity of lungs (diffusion of gases from blood to lungs (CO_2) and lungs to blood (O_2). It measures the amount of carbon dioxide and oxygen gases crossing membrane of air sacs per minute. It is carried out to calculate the arterial amount of different gases in the body and how efficiently lung transfers very small amount of carbon monoxide (CO) into the blood stream. Carbon monoxide diffusing capacity (also called transfer factor, or TF), which measures how well your lungs transfer a small amount of carbon monoxide (CO) into the blood. Two different methods are used for this test. If the single-breath or breath-holding method is used, you will take a breath of air containing a very small amount of carbon monoxide from a container while measurements are taken. In the steady-state method, you will breathe air containing a very small amount of carbon monoxide from a container. The amount of carbon monoxide in the breath you exhale is then measured. Diffusing capacity provides an estimate of how well a gas is able to move from your lungs into your blood.

4.2.5.3 Body plethysmography

This test is performed to measure the TLC (Total lung capacity) of the patient. The patient is allowed to sit in a closed chamber called as plethysmograph and allowed to breathe out in a mouth piece and the other end is joined to the spirogram which will measure the flow and interpreted. Body plethysmography is particularly appropriate for patients who have air spaces within the lung that do not communicate with the bronchial tree. In these individuals, gas dilution methods of measurement would give an erroneously low volume reading.

There are two types of plethysmographs: a) Flow, b) Pressure.

(a) In *flow plethysmography*, airway resistance is measured by two maneuvers. The patient first pants while the mouth shutter is open to allow flow changes to be measured. Then, the mouth shutter closes at the patient's end expiratory or FRC level and the patient continues panting while maintaining an open glottis. This provides a measure of the driving pressure used to move air into the lungs.

(b) *Pressure plethysmographs* are usually measured at the end-expiratory level and are then equal to FRC. The patient sits in the box, which has the pressure transducer in the wall of the device, and breathes through a mouthpiece connected to a device that contains an electronic shutter and a differential pressure pneumotachometer. The mouth pressure and box pressure changes that are measured during tidal breathing and panting maneuvers which are performed during the test by the patient at the end of expiration are sent to a microprocessor unit that calculates thoracic gas volume.

4.2.5.4 Inhalational challenge test

This test is performed to check that the patient is stimulated by what type of allergen and in what quantity. It is also called as *proactive studies*. For this the patient is made to inhale the allergen as an inhaler using nebulizer. It is slightly inhaled by the patient followed by spirometery at regular intervals of time. Also histamines and methacholines are induced in the body at regular intervals of time. In very rare cases, bronchospasm may occur but it is immediately treated with effective bronchodilators. It is normally employed in the diagnosis of occupational rhinitis.

4.2.5.5 Excessive stress test

This test is performed to check how much sudden and continuous stress lung has the capacity to tolerate. For this patient is made to do a stressful exercise continuously. After some interval of time spirometery is done.

4.2.6 Estimation of Blood Pressure

Blood pressure is basically a pressure exerted by the blood on the walls of artery. This pressure is produced by the blood pumping action of heart. Two types of pressure is exerted by the blood: systolic and diastolic. Systolic pressure is always higher than the diastolic pressure.

(a) **The systolic pressure** is the maximum pressure in an artery at the moment when the heart is beating and pumping blood through the body.

(b) **The diastolic pressure** is the lowest pressure in an artery in the moments between beats when the heart is resting.

Blood pressure varies from individual to individual and is dependant upon a number of factors, such as age and weight, physical condition, or gender. The classic normal reading for an adult between the ages of 18 and 45 is 120/80. Remember, only your physician is qualified to determine whether the readings you obtain are normal for you. There are three methods to measuring blood pressure

(i) **Palpatory method**: study of pulses from wrist, neck etc. It is done only if proper instruments are not available or in case of emergency.

(ii) **Oscillatory method**: This method is used in digital meters and involves the study of oscillations produced due to blood.

(iii) **Ausculatory method**: It is done by applying pressure over the artery and to stop the blood and then study the blood pressure by releasing the pressure slowly. Based on last two methods there are certain devices to measure B.P. These include:

4.2.6.1 Mercury sphygmomanometer

This device is based on the auscultatory method of blood pressure determination. The device consists of mercury column, cuff, pressure pump and a stethoscope. To take a blood pressure reading, you need to be relaxed and comfortably seated, with your arm well supported. Alternatively, you can lie on an examination couch.

- A cuff that inflates is wrapped around your upper arm and kept in place with Velcro. A tube leads out of the cuff to a rubber bulb.

- Another tube leads from the cuff to a reservoir of mercury at the bottom of a vertical glass column. Whatever pressure is in the cuff is shown on the mercury column. The mercury is held within a sealed system – only air travels in the rubber tubing and the cuff.

- Air is then blown into the cuff and increasing pressure and tightening is felt on the upper arm.

- The doctor puts a stethoscope to your arm and listens to the pulse while the air is slowly let out again.

- The systolic pressure is measured when the doctor first hears the pulse.

- This sound will slowly become more distant and finally disappear.

- The diastolic pressure is measured from the moment the doctor is unable to hear the sound of the pulse.

- The blood pressure is measured in terms of millimeters of mercury (mmHg).

It is highly simple and the oldest method and even do not need any calibration.

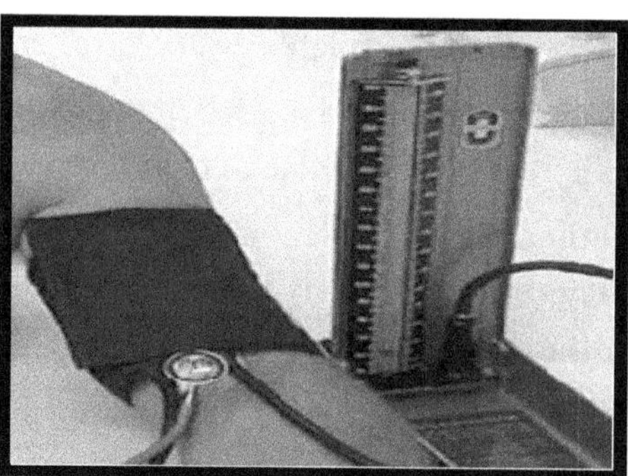

Fig. 4.4 Measurement of Blood Pressure

4.2.6.2 Finger monitors

These are digital monitors. They have small cuff that can be tied around the finger. After few seconds, the monitor automatically shows reading. Such devices need proper calibration before usage.

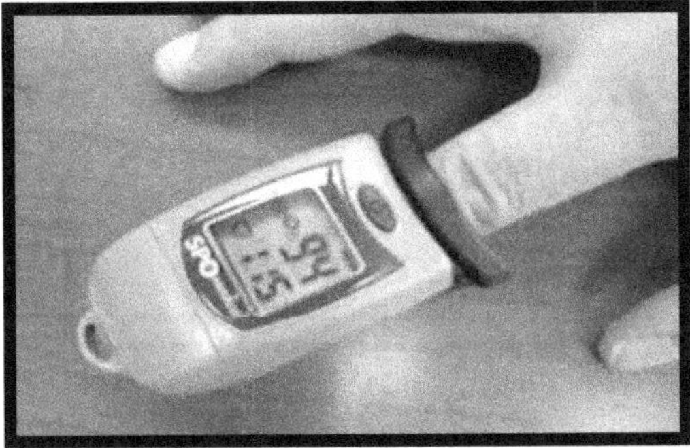

Fig. 4.5 Finger Monitor

4.2.6.3 Digital monitors

These are digital monitors which can be cuff tied on the upper elbow region and then the monitor studies the oscillations produced in the blood vessel due to pulsary moments of the blood. These monitors works on oscillometric technique. These monitors can be used for overweight and obese patients. They also require frequent calibration.

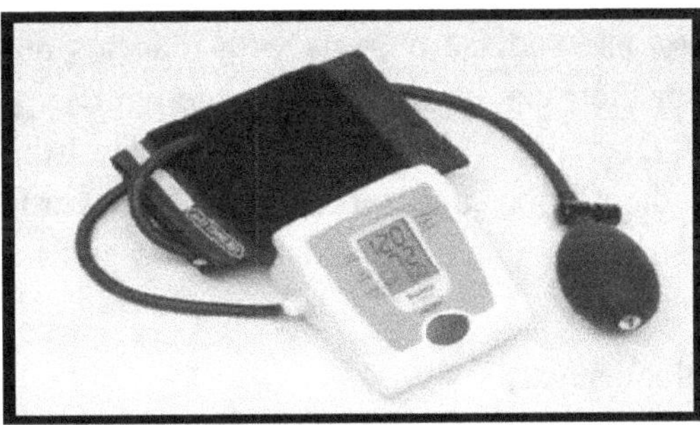

Fig. 4.6 Digital monitor

4.2.6.4 Aneroid sphygmomanometer

They are similar to mercury sphygmomanometer but have dial to be read. They are comparatively less expensive, portable and light in weight. It also requires calibration prior to its use.

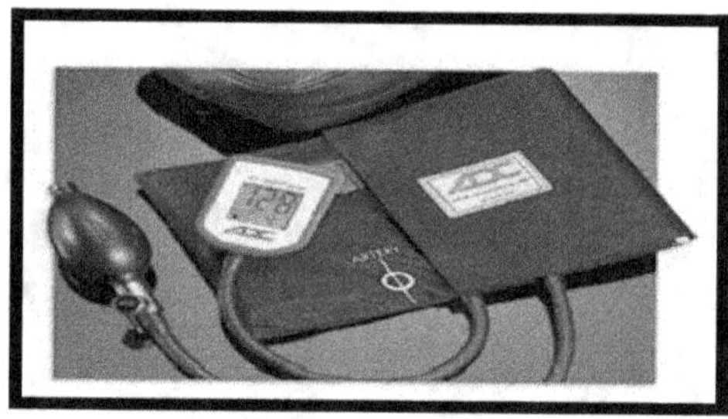

Fig. 4.7 Aneroid Sphygmanometer

4.2.7 Blood Glucose Monitoring

Blood glucose monitoring is a way of testing the concentration of glucose in the blood (glycemia). Particularly important in the care of diabetes mellitus, a blood glucose test is performed by piercing the skin (typically, on the finger) to draw blood, then applying the blood to a chemically active disposable 'test-strip'. Different manufacturers use different technology, but most systems measure an electrical characteristic, and use this to determine the glucose level in the blood.

Healthcare professionals advise patients with diabetes on the appropriate monitoring regime for their condition. Most people with Type 2 diabetes test at least once per day. Diabetics who use insulin (all Type 1 diabetes and many Type 2s) usually test their blood sugar more often (3 to 10 times per day), both to assess the effectiveness of their prior insulin dose and to help determine their next insulin dose.

Normal Results of Blood sugar:

- Before meals: 70 - 130 milligrams per deciliter (mg/dL)
- After meals: Less than 180 mg/dL

Values can vary depending on physical activity, meals, and insulin administration. Normal value ranges may vary slightly among different laboratories. The various techniques employed for the estimation of level of glucose in blood include:

1. Benedict's Test
2. Glucometers
3. Using GOD/POD (Glucose Oxidase Peroxidase) test.

4.2.7.1 Digital glucometers/ blood glucose meters

A blood glucose meter is an electronic device for measuring the blood glucose level. A relatively small drop of blood is placed on a disposable test strip which interfaces with a digital meter. Within several seconds, the level of blood glucose will be shown on the digital display.

Needing only a small drop of blood for the meter means that the pain associated with testing is reduced and the compliance of diabetic people to their testing regimens is improved. Although the cost of using blood glucose meters seems high, it is believed to be a cost benefit relative to the avoided medical costs of the complications of diabetes.

4.2.7.2 Recent and welcome advances include

- *'alternate site testing'*, the use of blood drops for from other places than the finger, usually the palm or forearm. This alternate site testing uses the same test strips and meter, is practically pain free, and gives the real estate on the finger tips a needed break if they become sore. The disadvantage of this technique is that there is usually less blood flow to alternate sites, which prevents the reading from being accurate when the blood sugar level is changing.

- *'no coding' systems*. Older systems required 'coding' of the strips to the meter. This carried a risk of 'miscoding', which can lead to inaccurate results. Two approaches have resulted systems that no longer require coding. Some systems are 'autocoded', where technology is used to code each strip to the meter. And some are manufactured to a 'single code', thereby avoiding the risk of miscoding.

- *'multi-test' systems*. Some systems use a cartridge or a disc containing multiple test strips. This has the advantage that the user doesn't have to load individual strips each time, which is convenient and can enable quicker testing.

- *'downloadable' meters*. Most newer systems come with software that allows the user to download meter results to a computer. This information can then be used, together with health care professional guidance, to enhance and improve diabetes management. The meters usually require a connection cable, unless they are designed to work wirelessly with an insulin pump, or are designed to plug directly into the computer.

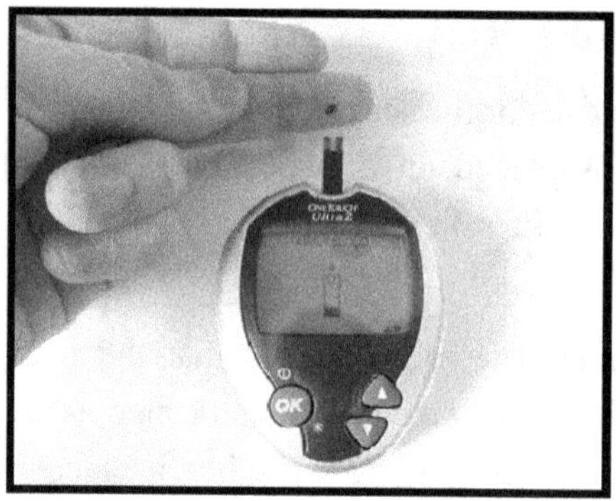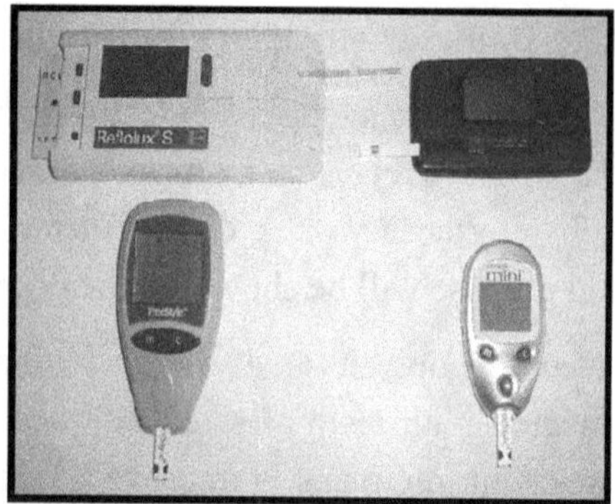

Fig. 4.8 Various types of Blood Glucose Meters

Colorimetric Analysis: This test is known to provide accurate laboratory test results. Very commonly used analytical methods include

4.2.7.3 GOD-POD test

This test is also called as glucose oxidase-peroxidase test. In this test, D-glucose of a sample reacts with water and oxygen in the presence of enzyme 'glucose peroxidase'. The reaction takes place and D-glucose gets converted into D-gluconic acid.

Hydrogen peroxide formed in the reaction-1, in the presence of enzyme peroxidase (POD) oxidizes phenol which combines with 4-aminio antipyrine (4-AMP) to produce a red or pink colored quinone dye. The intensity of color is proportional to glucose concentration in the sample. The final color is stable only for 24 hours. The test is carried in three tubes marked as Blank (B), Standard (S) and Test (T). After formation of dye, standard and test are studied against blank on photo-colorimeter with green filter or on spectrophotometer at 505 nm. Then the readings are substituted in the following formula to estimate the glucose concentration.

$$\text{D-Glucose} + H_2O_2 \xrightarrow{\text{Glucose Oxidase}} \text{D-Glucose Acid} + H_2O_2$$

$$2H_2O_2 + \text{4-aminoantipyrine} + \text{Phenol} \xrightarrow{\text{Peroxidase}} \text{Red Quinone dye} + 4H_2O$$

$$\text{Glucose in mg \%} = \frac{\text{Absorbance of test}}{\text{Absorbance of standard}} \times 100$$

4.2.7.4 Nelson and somogyi's method

The protein free sample is boiled with alkaline copper tartarate. The cupric ions are reduced by the glucose to cuprous ions.

$$\text{Glucose} + Cu^{3+} \xrightarrow{\text{Boil}} Cu^{2+}$$

$$Cu^{2+} \xrightarrow{\text{Arseno–molybdic acid}} \text{Arsenomolybdous acid (red)}$$

Cuprous ions in turn forms arsenomolybdous acid from arsenomolybdic acid which is red in color and the extent of the glucose present is measured colorimetrically.

In the first step, glucose (or a reducing sugar) is oxidised using a solution of Cu (II) ion which in the process is reduced to Cu (I). In the second step the Cu (I) ions are then oxidised back to Cu (II) using a colourless hetero-polymolybdate complex, which is, in the process, reduced to give the characteristic blue colour. Finally the absorption of the hetero-poly molybdenum blue is measured using a colorimeter and compared to standards prepared from reacting sugar solutions of known concentration, to determine the amount of reducing-sugar present.

The Somogyi-Nelson method uses an arsenomolybdate complex formed by the reaction of ammonium molybdate with sodium arsenate.

4.2.8 Evaluation of Blood Cholesterol

Cholesterol accounts for almost all of the sterol in plasma. It exists as a mixture of unesterified (30 to 40 %) and esterified (60 to 70 %) forms. The proportion of the two forms is constant within and between normal individuals. Various adaptations of the colorimetric and the enzymatic assays can use for cholesterol estimation. Most diagnostic and the research laboratories use the enzymatic assay method. However, the following experiment uses the chemical (colorimetric) method to determine the plasma cholesterol level.

The cholesterol test determines patient total cholesterol (TC), low density lipoproteins (LDL) and high density lipoproteins (HDL) and triglycerides.

(i) Some test provides the patients only with TC level whereas other provides a full lipid profile (TC, HDL, LDL and triglycerides etc.)

(ii) Some cholesterol kits are a single use test in which patients apply a blood sample on collecting card, which is mailed to the laboratory for evaluation. The measurement of amount of cholesterol is determined by the color chart which is provided with the test.

(iii) Colorimetric analysis:

    (a) Reusable cholesterol monitors are available and they use reflectance photometery technology to convert the color changes produced into a rapidly on a liquid crystal display screen.

    (b) Chemical reaction involves (it contains ferric perchlorate ethyl acetate and sulphuric acid)

Cholesterol + Cholesterol reagent $\longrightarrow$ Produces lavender colored complex
(sample)

    (c) Principle: This test is also called as ZAK test.

This reddish purple color complex is measured calorimetrically.

Serum   + Ferric chloride acetic acid reagent $\longrightarrow$ Reddish purple
(sample-protein free)   colored complex

Interpretation: Serum cholesterol varies from 150-240 mg/100ml of blood in a healthy adult.

4.2.9 Health Related Quality of Life (HRQL)

Although quality of life focuses on all aspects of life, HRQL focuses on patient's non clinical information such as functional status, perception of health and other health outcomes that are directly affected by the health status. Various techniques for carrying out HRQL includes:

1. Questionnaire Technique
2. Telephone Interviews
2. Face to face interview
4. Mail-in-survey.

Questionnaire technique can also be divided in general health status instruments like SF-36, SF-10 are for children's, SF-8 for health services. Telephonic and face to face interviews are for verbal and side by side non-verbal aspects also are very helpful for the same.

HEALTH EDUCATION

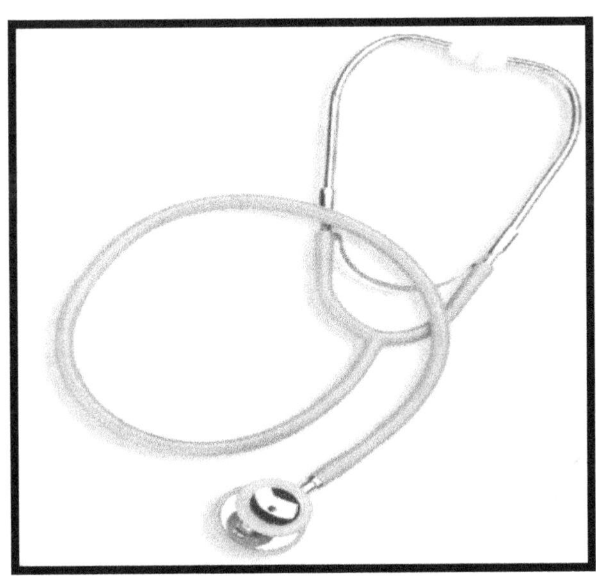

5.1 HEALTH EDUCATION

5.1.1 WHO Definition of Health

WHO since its endorsement on 7th April 1948 is the only and the most efficient technical and professional body concerned with international public health issues.

WHO constitution describes health as "state of complete physical, mental and social well-being and not only merely the absence of disease or infirmity". Its overall objective is the attainment by all peoples of the highest possible levels of health. Efforts of WHO has come up with several achievements in the field of health. As in this century, there were significantly gains in life expectancy of 20-40 years worldwide.

The organization has to consider the diversity of health challenge in order to develop strategies and programs to meet the needs of its member states and to achieve better health for all.

5.1.2 Objectives of World Health Organization

1. Providing guidance and advocacy for health by ethics, EBM etc.
2. Stimulation of appropriate health technology.
3. Setting global norms and standards.
4. Information management.
5. Negotiation and sustenance of national and global partnership.
6. Cooperation to Government in strengthening NHPs.

5.2 HEALTH PROMOTION

Health promotion is about providing services that improve health of individual and communities finally resulting in empowerment of them to so that they have increased control over their own health.

5.2.1 Classification of Health Promotion Activities

Classification of Health Promotion Activities conducted by pharmacist

1. Promotion of health and well-being (nutrition, physical activity etc.).
2. Identification of illness (screening and detection of diseases).

3. Prevention of illness (smoking cessation, immunization, travel health etc.).

4. Maintenance of health for those with chronic diseases like asthma, hypertension etc.

All these health promotion activities results in:

(a) Total compliance of individual at one end.

(b) Varying degree of compliance.

(c) Total non-compliance.

5.2.2 Models of Health Promotion

5.2.2.1 Medical approach

This approach aims for freedom from medically defined diseases like diabetes, cancers etc. through medical investigation techniques like immunization, screening etc.

5.2.2.2 Behavioral change

This approach aims at alteration of attitude and behavior so that changed behavior is conducive to freedom from disease and healthy life style by advising them to consume alcohol sensibly, stop smoking etc.

5.2.2.3 Education approach

This approach aims to provide information so that individuals have knowledge and understanding about health issues by health promotion leaflets, educational programs, national campaigns etc.

5.2.2.4 Patient-centered approach

This includes empower individuals to make their own decisions.

5.2.2.5 Patient-centered approach

This approach aims at self-empowerment of individuals to make them enable to have control on their health destinies.

5.2.2.6 Societal change

Includes bringing a change in society making environment a better living place such as making smoking socially unacceptable and making the use of condoms acceptable in the society.

5.2.3 Role of Pharmacists

5.2.3.1 Sales of goods other than medicines

For example, children toothpaste, ovulating testing kit and health promotion activities include like distribution of leaflets on oral health care, various diseases like diabetes, AIDS, hypertension etc. to create more awareness among general public.

5.2.3.2 Sales of medicine

Especially OTC medications provide the aliment of the concerned person and health promotion activity can be provided likely as all purchases of nicotine replacement therapy should be encouraged at smoking cessations.

5.2.3.3 Prescription medicines

Prescription medicines give an indication of illness suffered by the patients or side effects of medicines necessitate giving advice as foot care advice to diabetic patients and reduced sodium intake for patients with conditions like hypertension.

5.2.3.4 Responding to symptoms

Responding to symptoms by pharmacist lead to promotion of health as diarrhoea and scurvy symptoms are common with travellers. The various provisions of health promotion materials include leaflets, books and pamphlets etc.

5.3   HEALTH CARE FOR PREGNANT WOMEN

Many of the pregnant women undergo the state of dilemma when drugs are to be used by them and on certain occasions it becomes quite difficult to take decision whether to go for Prescription drugs or Non Prescription Drugs (NPDs). For various reasons, study on proper use of the drugs during human pregnancy is few and prescribing of drugs during pregnancy is more or less arbitrary rather than rational. Most of the drugs taken by the pregnant women can cross the placenta and exert their pharmacological and teratogenic effects on the developing embryo/fetus. So, while taking medication during pregnancy women should observe utmost care and precautions.

5.3.1 Factors Affecting Placental Drug Transfer

I   Physicochemical Factors

   (i) *Lipid solubility*: Lipophilic drugs tend to diffuse readily across the placenta and enter the fetus circulation. An example is Thiopental, which is commonly used for cesarean sections. Thiopental crosses the placenta immediately and produces sedation or apnea in the newborn infant.

   (ii) *Molecular size*: Drugs with molecular weight of 250-500 Da can cross the placenta easily depending upon their lipid solubility and degree of ionization.

   (iii) *Placental transporter*: During the last decade, increasing number of drug transporters has been identified. P-glycoprotein is one such transporter encoded by M-D-R1G pumps drug back into the maternal circulation. Inhibition of these transporters may cause drug accumulation in the fetus.

   (iv) *Protein binding*: Due to increased lipophilicity, drugs tend to bind with the body tissues and proteins which ultimately affects the fetus e.g. Sulfonamides, barbiturates, phenytoin and local anesthetic agents.

   (v) *Placental and fetal drug metabolism*: Two important mechanisms protects the fetus from drugs in maternal circulation:

   (a) Placenta itself acts as semi permeable barrier and also as a site of metabolism of some drugs e.g. Pentobarbital is metabolized via aromatic oxidation reaction.

   (b) Drugs that cross the placenta enter the fetal circulation via the umbilical vein. About 40-60% of umbilical venous blood flow enters the fetal liver. The remainder bypasses the liver and enters the general fetal circulation.

II The rate at which the drug crosses the placenta and amount of the drug reaching the fetus.

III The duration of exposure to drug.

IV Distribution characteristics in different fetal tissues.

V The stage of placental and fetal development at the time of exposure to the drug.

VI The effects of drugs used in combination.

In order to provide safe and effective drug therapy to such category of patients, it is important to gain knowledge of the pharmacokinetic and pharmacodynamic properties of each drug and the effect of development on its disposition. The chronological detail of pediatric patients has been shown in Table 5.1.

Table 5.1 Chronological time.

S. No.	Period /Duration between	Terminology
1.	Conception and Birth	Post-Conceptional age/Gestational age
2.	Birth and 4 weeks	Neonate
3.	4 weeks to 1 year	Infant
4.	1 year to 13 years	Child
5.	13 years to 18 years	Adolescence

The pregnant women is perhaps the last true therapeutic orphan because of the ethical, medico-legal and fetal safety concerns regarding pregnant women, few pharmacokinetic, pharmacodynamic and clinical trials are conducted during pregnancy. The risk most often considered is the fetal risk of teratogenesis or drug-induced malformation.

Teratogenic defects: Any birth defect either morphological, biochemical or behavioral induced at any stage of pregnancy and detected at birth or later in life called as teratogenic effects and agents inducing them called as teratogens and process called as teratogenicity.

5.3.2 Health Care in Pregnant and Breast Feeding Woman

Pregnant and breast feeding women are posing the most critical situations as predicted by medicos and pharmacist for pharmacotherapy. In fact, pregnant woman is the last true therapeutic orphan as she provides way to both twice therapy and risk. Various drugs can cause teratogenic effects during pregnancy like:

Table 5.2 Few of the medications exhibiting teratogenic effects.

Drug	*Effect*
Thalidomide	Phocomelia (limb shortening)
Alcohol	Facial dysmorphogenesis, growth and mental retardation
Tetracycline	Bone deposits, teeth discoloration
Coumadin	Nasal hypoplasia, optic atrophy
Folic acid	Abortion, microcephaly
Diazepam	Leads to neonatal dependence

A lot of care is required to be taken of a pregnant woman as drugs penetrate the placenta and reach the fetus. Following are the points for care-

5.3.2.1 Planning for pregnancy

Woman should be made both mentally and emotionally prepared for pregnancy. Pathological condition of them should be strong and satisfactory.

5.3.2.2 Proper pathological monitoring

Should be carried out for detection of diseases like epilepsy that must be cured by mono-therapy so that maternal and fetal risk can be prevented by proper medication.

5.3.2.3 Counseling

The pregnant women should be adequately counseled about the drugs used by them. They should be given counseling regarding exercise, nutrition and about life-style which they must follow to avert diseases of fetus.

5.3.2.4 Detection of fetus abnormality

If it is predicted during early period of pregnancy then it can be terminated or proper therapy can be provided.

5.3.3 Precautions While Prescribing/Administering Drugs to a Pregnant Woman

- Treat minor aliments without drugs.

- If a drug must be prescribed, it should be one, which is known to be safe during pregnancy.

- Advice the patients that absolute safety of the fetus cannot be guaranteed even by not prescribing any drug to woman between the age of 15-45. Therefore do not sacrifice the mother's interest for the sake of the fetus.

- Prefer a drug, which has been in use for a long period of time to newly introduced drugs, as the safety of the latter for fetus is not likely to be known completely.

- Adjust the dose of the drug depending on the pregnant stage. With most drugs, it is generally at the lower end of the therapeutic range. However, because of pharmacokinetic factors (increased body weight, more rapid clearance); the dose of certain drugs such as lithium, digoxin and phenytoin is likely to be higher than in the non-pregnant state in some women.

5.3.4 Care for Nursing Mother

One of the many objectives of healthy people 2010 is to have 75% of mothers initiating breast-feeding, 50% of mothers breast-feeding for the first six months, and 25% of mothers breast-feeding for the first 12 months. It is important for pharmacists to understand the effects of OTC medications in women who are breast-feeding in order to make appropriate recommendations. It is very much ethical and justified on part of the pharmacist to make the breast feeding mothers aware and familiarize with the probable unwanted side effects associated with the OTC medications.

5.3.5 Transfer of Drugs into Breast Milk

Most medications will transfer into breast milk; however, the degree of transfer depends on several factors. Drugs may transfer into milk if they attain high concentrations in maternal plasma, have a low molecular weight (<500 Da), are low in protein binding, and are lipid soluble. During the first week of breast-feeding, when colostrum is produced, there are large gaps between the alveolar cells that enhance the passage of drugs into milk.

However, the quantity of milk produced at this time is low (< 30 to 100 ml/day), so the absolute dose transferred is minimal. After the first week, the presence of prolactin closes the gaps, reducing the entry of most maternal drugs and other substances into the milk compartment.

Various safety considerations for using medications while breast-feeding include

(a) Choosing drugs with short half-lives, high protein binding, low oral bioavailability or high molecular weight.

(b) To decrease infant exposure to the drug or taking the medication immediately after breast-feeding and avoiding long-acting formulations.

(c) A clinician should choose a medication with published safety data rather than a newly introduced medication.

(d) The most important thing to remember when you are breast-feeding is that practically everything that goes into your body also goes into your milk. Therefore, before you eat, drink or take an over the counter or prescribed medication you should consider how it will affect your child and what would be the effect of medication on lactation.

5.3.6 Pre-Administration Considerations

Consider not only safety of the drug in question, but also the possibility that there may be a safer alternative or drug of choice in breast-feeding. Avoid new drugs if a therapeutically equivalent alternative that has been more widely used is available.

Background information

- Is the mother breast-feeding and has she already taken a medicine (retrospective enquiry)?

- Is the mother breast-feeding and want to take a medicine (prospective enquiry)?

- Is the mother taking a medicine and want to breast-feed (prospective enquiry)?

- What is the baby's age, including gestational age?

- Does the baby have any medical problems?

- What medication is the mother taking or wants to take?

- What are the doses and dosage frequency?

- What is the indication for the medication?

- Has the mother taken any of the drugs during the pregnancy?

5.4 HEALTH CARE OF GERIATRIC PATIENTS

Geriatric is the branch of general medicine concerned with the clinical, preventive, remedial and social aspects of illness in the elderly. The term elderly generally refers to patients aged 60 years and above. Older people tend to have more long-term, chronic illnesses such as arthritis, diabetes, high blood pressure and heart disease than younger people, well known characteristics of geriatric patients.

It is well documented that people aged 60 and older are the largest consumers of prescription and over-the-counter (OTC) medicines than any other age group, according to the National Institute on Aging. Recent estimates show that adults age 60 and older take an average of five prescription medications each day. In 1997, it was found that 87% of older individuals (mean age 74.5 years) reported regular use of at least one over-the-counter (OTC) medication, and 5.7% were taking five or more OTC medications daily. Given the recent rise in use of nutraceuticals, these figures are likely to be underestimated.

The Food and Drug Administration (FDA) is working to make drugs safer for older people, who consume a large share of the nation's medications. People over age 65 buy 30% of all prescription drugs and 40% of all OTC drugs. There has been consistent concern that the number of medications taken by older adult patients can lead to increase in disability and the potential for life-threatening illness. Furthermore, it is important to consider specifically the effects of medications acting on central nervous system because older adults commonly use them and moreover the brain is the most vulnerable part of human systems.

Another contributor to medication misadventures is the increase in the use of non-prescription or OTC drugs, especially by the elderly. Additionally, herbal and nutritional supplements and other alternative remedies are becoming part of the culture of health and wellness. Many of these products have not been proven effective, much less safe. Over-the-counter drugs, health food products and alternative products are widely available now a days.

The elderly, who use 40% of all non-prescription products, consider them to be safe and relatively innocuous. Since the mid-1980s, a large number of prescription drugs have been moved from prescription-only to over-the-counter status, and more are on the way. Patients now have access to effective nonprescription drugs, many of which produce physiologic responses that interact with prescription medications. The prevailing attitude is that OTC products can be used nonchalantly because they are not as powerful as prescription medications.

Older people who experience dizziness, constipation, stomach upset, sleep changes, diarrhoea, blurred vision, mood changes, rashes, or other symptoms after taking a drug should call their doctors. The following suggestions may also help:

- Make sure you tell your doctor and pharmacist about all the medicines you take, including prescription and non-prescription medicines, vitamins, and herbal supplements. You may sometimes have more than one doctor, each prescribing different medicines. Make sure they all know what the others are prescribing, and ask one doctor to coordinate your drugs.

- Get all your prescriptions filled at one pharmacy. Your pharmacist can serve as a central point to maintain a list of all your medicines, and can screen for drug interactions to avoid harmful situations.

- Tell your doctor if you are allergic to any medicines.

- Keep track of side effects. New symptoms may not be from old age but from the drug you're taking.

- Learn about your drugs. Find out as much as you can by asking questions and reading the package inserts. Both your doctor and pharmacist should alert you about the possible drug interactions, adverse and side effects, dose, dosage regimen etc.

- Have your doctor reviewed your drugs? If you take a number of drugs, take them all with you on a doctor's visit.

- Follow directions. Read the label every time you take the medication to prevent mistakes, and be sure you understand the timing, dose prescribed, and how long to take it. Ask a pharmacist for possible food-drug interactions. Some drugs are better absorbed with certain foods, and some drugs shouldn't be taken with certain foods.

- Don't forget to take your medicines. Use a memory aid like a calendar, pillbox, or your own system. Whatever works for you is best to help you.

5.4.1 OTC Medications: Strategies to be Adopted by Elderly Patients

(i) Arthritis, poor eyesight, and memory lapses can make it difficult for some older people to take their medications correctly. Studies have shown that between 40% and 75% of older people don't take their medications at the right time or in the right amount.

(ii) A number of strategies can make taking medication easier. Patients with arthritis can ask the pharmacist for an oversized, easy-to-open bottle. For easier reading, ask for large-type labels. If those are not available, use a magnifying glass and read the label under bright light.

(iii) Invent a system to remember medication. Even younger people have trouble remembering several medications two or three times a day, with and without food. Devise a plan that fits your daily schedule. Some people use meals or bedtime as clues for remembering drugs. Others use charts, calendars, and special weekly pillboxes, and techniques such as turning medicine bottles upside down, to help them know at a glance if they have taken the medication.

(iv) Drug-taking routines should take into account whether the medication works best on an empty or full stomach and whether the doses are spaced properly. To simplify drug taking, always ask for the easiest dosing schedule that's available for the drug you've been prescribed for example just once or twice a day.

(v) Older people with serious memory impairments require assistance from family members or professionals. Adult day care, supervised living facilities, and home health nurses can provide assistance with drugs.

5.5 HEALTH CARE FOR PEDIATRICS

The pediatric population comprises 20-25% of the total world population, and numerous acute and chronic diseases can affect this sub-population. Premature neonates have poorly developed organ functions and are at higher risk of eliciting unexpected toxicity or poor clinical response from suboptimal dosage regimens of drug due to altered pharmacokinetics or dosage requirement in the population. The sulfanilamide and thalidomide tragedies (deaths due to sulfanilamide elixir, and birth defects among the newborns from mothers who had used thalidomide for motion sickness) have focused the attention of all concerned and the Government is being forced to put strict controls and requirements for drug approval in case of pediatric patients.

Numerous studies over the last three decades have shown that pediatric patients are unique in many ways. It is necessary to understand that children are not 'miniature adults'; the adult doses, scaled down based on body weights may not be safe or effective in the pediatric population. As neonates develop into infants and young adolescents, a number of physiological changes occur in their body composition e.g. change in water, fat, plasma proteins, and hormonal composition in the body that influence drug disposition and dosage requirements. The unique aspects of pediatric drug therapy has to be taken into consideration while deciding for OTC therapy in case of pediatric patients. Such unique aspects may be listed as –

(i)   They require different doses per kilogram of body weight than adults due to differences in the pharmacokinetics, pharmacodynamics and various other factors.

(ii)   Pediatric patients below six years of age may need extemporaneously prepared dosage forms e.g. oral suspensions due to their inability to swallow tablets or capsules and the fact that doses are not fixed based on body weights.

(iii)   Patients are dependent on parents or caregivers to receive optimal drug therapy.

(iv)   The social and economic status of parents directly influences the care they can offer to their children.

(v)   Certain intrinsic factors such as gender, race, heredity and inherited diseases and extrinsic factors such as acquired diseases, diet, and prior exposure to drug therapy may change drug disposition in the pediatric patients.

(vi)   FDA is working on changing the labels of over-the-counter medications to make them more eye-catching, easier to read, and consumer-friendly. For prescription drugs, FDA took measures in December 1994 to provide more information to health-care providers about use of those products in children.

(vii)   The agency now lets prescription drug manufacturers make more focus on pediatric labeling, the data of which is extrapolated from adequate and well-controlled adult studies, together with other information about safety and dosing in children. This is allowed as long as the agency concludes that the course of the disease and the drug's effects are sufficiently similar in children and adults.

(viii)   Presently, most prescription drugs do not contain pediatric doses on their labels. A 1979 regulation required full clinical trials in children as the basis for pediatric labeling. Doctors who need to prescribe those drugs to children do so based on their own experience and reports in medical literature. The new regulations will give health-care providers more information to prescribe medicine for children safely.

(ix)   In addition, FDA is taking steps to increase the numbers of drugs being tested in children. The goal of FDA's changes is to ensure that whenever a child receives medication, it is as safe and effective as possible.

5.6   COMMUNICABLE DISEASES

These are the infectious diseases in which causative organism may pass from person to person directly or indirectly example typhoid, malaria, AIDS, dysentery etc.

5.6.1 Modes of Transmission

(a)   Contacts, carriers and convalescents are the main modes of transmission of communicable diseases. Contacts and carriers are the major contributors.

(b)   Clothes, furniture, books, utensils etc. spread the diseases, coming in contact with these belongings of patient transfers the infection.

(c)   Reuse of used medico-instruments like injections, needles etc. also cause spread of disease as infected instruments inculcate causative microbes.

(d)   Infected transfusions of blood and blood related substance and also of organs can also result in infections which are highly fatal.

(e)   Lack of hygiene like using the same toilets, towels as used by the patient can transfer the disease.

5.6.2 Preventive Measures

(a)   *Notification to public:* Various advertisements, pamphlets should be distributed to public especially to rural masses in order to clarify their doubts.

(b) *Patient isolation* is must. Restriction should be exercised on visitors to places which are affected by patients. After nursing hands should be properly washed.

(c) *Proper sanitation* includes safe water supply, proper disposal of excreta and waste and proper sanitation facilities.

(d) *Control on carriers* is required to prevent the diseases from becoming epidemic. Flies and mosquitoes can be controlled by employing proper insecticides.

(e) *Proper precautions and use of contraceptive devices* to prevent sexually transmitted diseases and reuse of the used micro-devices should be avoided.

5.7 NUTRITION

Any substance which is digested, absorbed and utilized to promote body functions called nutrients e.g. fFats, carbohydrates, proteins, vitamins and minerals etc.

Balanced diet is the diet which contains all the essential nutrients in adequate quantities according to sex, age, occupation and pathological conditions of an individual.

Nutrition science investigates the metabolic and physiological responses of the body to diet. With advances in the fields of molecular biology, biochemistry, and genetics, the study of nutrition is increasingly concerned with metabolism and metabolic pathways: the sequences of biochemical steps through which substances in living things change from one form to another.

Nitrogen is needed by animals to build proteins. Carnivore and herbivore diets vary in their source of nitrogen, which is a limiting nutrient for both. Herbivores consume plants to get nitrogen and carnivores consume other animals to obtain nitrogen. Nitrogen is a common element in the atmosphere but exists in a state that is not usable by most living organisms. Certain fungi and bacteria are able to convert atmospheric nitrogen into a form plants can adsorb and utilize.

The human body contains chemical compounds, such as water, carbohydrates (sugar, starch, and fiber), amino acids (in proteins), fatty acids (in lipids), and nucleic acids (DNA and RNA). These compounds in turn consist of elements such as carbon, hydrogen, oxygen, nitrogen, phosphorus, calcium, iron, zinc, magnesium, manganese, and so on. All of these chemical compounds and elements occur in various forms and combinations (e.g., hormones, vitamins, phospholipids, hydroxyapatite), both in the human body and in the plant and animal organisms that humans eat.

The human body consists of elements and compounds ingested, digested, absorbed, and circulated through the bloodstream to feed the cells of the body. Except in the unborn fetus, which receives processed nutrients from the mother, the digestive system is the first system involved in breaking down food prior to further digestion. Digestive juices, excreted into the lumen of the gastrointestinal tract, break chemical bonds in ingested molecules, and modulate their conformations and energy states. Though some molecules are absorbed into the bloodstream unchanged, digestive processes release them from the matrix of foods. Unabsorbed matter, along with some waste products of metabolism, is eliminated from the body in the feces.

Studies of nutritional status must take into account the state of the body before and after experiments, as well as the chemical composition of the whole diet and of all material excreted and eliminated from the body (in urine and feces). Comparing the food to the waste can help determine the specific compounds and elements absorbed and metabolized in the body. The effects of nutrients may only be discernible over an extended period, during which all food and waste must be analyzed. The number of variables involved in such experiments is high, making nutritional studies time-consuming and expensive.

In general, eating a wide variety of fresh, whole (unprocessed), foods has proven favorable for one's health compared to monotonous diets based on processed foods.

In particular, the consumption of whole-plant foods slows digestion and allows better absorption, and a more favorable balance of essential nutrients per Calorie, resulting in better management of cell growth, maintenance, and mitosis (cell division), as well as better regulation of appetite and blood sugar.

Regularly scheduled meals (every few hours) have also proven more wholesome than infrequent or haphazard ones, although a recent study has also linked more frequent meals with a higher risk of colon cancer in men.

There are six major classes of nutrients: carbohydrates, fats, minerals, protein, vitamins, and water.

These nutrient classes can be categorized as either macronutrients (needed in relatively large amounts) or macronutrients (needed in smaller quantities). The macronutrients include carbohydrates, fats, protein, and water. The micronutrients are minerals and vitamins.

The macronutrients (excluding water) provide structural material (amino acids from which proteins are built, and lipids from which cell membranes and some signaling molecules are built), energy. Some of the structural material can be used to generate energy internally, and in either case it is measured in Joules or kilocalories (often called "Calories" and written with a capital C to distinguish them from little 'c' calories). Carbohydrates and proteins provide 17 kJ approximately (4 kcal) of energy per gram, while fats provide 37 kJ (9 kcal) per gram, though the net energy from either depends on such factors as absorption and digestive effort, which vary substantially from instance to instance. Vitamins, minerals, fiber, and water do not provide energy, but are required for other reasons. A third class of dietary material, fiber (i.e., non-digestible material such as cellulose), is also required, for both mechanical and biochemical reasons, although the exact reasons remain unclear.

Molecules of carbohydrates and fats consist of carbon, hydrogen, and oxygen atoms. Carbohydrates range from simple monosaccharides (glucose, fructose, galactose) to complex polysaccharides (starch). Fats are triglycerides, made of assorted fatty acid monomers bound to glycerol backbone. Some fatty acids, but not all, are essential in the diet: they cannot be synthesized in the body. Protein molecules contain nitrogen atoms in addition to carbon, oxygen, and hydrogen. The fundamental components of protein are nitrogen-containing amino acids, some of which are essential in the sense that humans cannot make them internally. Some of the amino acids are convertible (with the expenditure of energy) to glucose and can be used for energy production just as ordinary glucose in a process known as gluconeogenesis. By breaking down existing protein, some glucose can be produced internally; the remaining amino acids are discarded, primarily as urea in urine. This occurs normally only during prolonged starvation.

Other micronutrients include antioxidants and phytochemicals, which are said to influence (or protect) some body systems. Their necessity is not as well established as in the case of, for instance, vitamins.

Most foods contain a mix of some or all of the nutrient classes, together with other substances, such as toxins of various sorts. Some nutrients can be stored internally (e.g., the fat soluble vitamins), while others are required more or less continuously. Poor health can be caused by a lack of required nutrients or, in extreme cases, too much of a required nutrient. For example, both salt and water (both absolutely required) will cause illness or even death in excessive amounts.

5.7.1 Carbohydrates

Carbohydrates include sugars, starches and fiber. They constitute a large part of foods such as rice, noodles, bread, and other grain-based products. Carbohydrates may be classified chemically as monosaccharides, disaccharides, or polysaccharides depending on the number of monomer (saccharide or sugar) units they contain. Monosaccharides, disaccharides, and polysaccharides contain one, two, and three or more sugar units, respectively.

Polysaccharides are often referred to as complex carbohydrates because they consist of long, sometimes branched chains of single sugar units. Mono- and disaccharides are called simple carbohydrates. Dietary advice frequently but erroneously suggests that complex carbohydrates are superior to simple because they take longer to digest and absorb. Simple carbohydrates, on the other hand, are said to cause a spike in blood glucose levels rapidly after ingestion. These traditional claims are false. In fact, many digestible polysaccharides are processed as rapidly and simple sugars in the human body. On the other hand some simple carbohydrates (fructose, for example) are processed in a different way and do not spike blood sugar. Thus the distinction between "complex" and "simple" does not predict the nutritional value or impact of carbohydrates. A better way of determining what effect particular foods may have on blood sugar and ultimately on health in general is the glycemic index.

Carbohydrates are not essential nutrients (with the likely exception of fiber), but are typically an important part of the human diet. While it would not be accurate to categorize all carbohydrates as "bad" nutritionally, some carbohydrate sources may well have deleterious effects on health, especially when consumed in large quantities. Highly processed carbohydrates (sugars and starches) as well as fructose consumed in large quantities have been implicated in negative health outcomes.

5.7.2 Fats

A molecule of dietary fat typically consists of several fatty acids (containing long chains of carbon and hydrogen atoms), bonded to a glycerol. They are typically found as triglycerides (three fatty acids attached to one glycerol backbone). Fats may be classified as saturated or unsaturated depending on the detailed structure of the fatty acids involved. Saturated fats have all of the carbon atoms in their fatty acid chains bonded to hydrogen atoms, whereas unsaturated fats have some of these carbon atoms double-bonded, so their molecules have relatively fewer hydrogen atoms than a saturated fatty acid of the same length.

Unsaturated fats may be further classified as monounsaturated (one double-bond) or polyunsaturated (many double-bonds). Furthermore, depending on the location of the double-bond in the fatty acid chain, unsaturated fatty acids are classified as omega-3 or omega-6 fatty acids. Trans fats are a type of unsaturated fat with trans-isomer bonds; these are rare in nature and in foods from natural sources; they are typically created in an industrial process called (partial) hydrogenation. There are nine kilocalories in each gram of fat.

Saturated fats (typically from animal sources) have been a staple in many world cultures for millennia. Unsaturated fats (e.g., vegetable oil) are considered healthier (citation needed), while trans fats are to be avoided. Saturated and some trans fats are typically solid at room temperature (such as butter or lard), while unsaturated fats are typically liquids (such as olive oil or flaxseed oil). Trans fats are very rare in nature, and have been shown to be highly detrimental to human health, but have properties useful in the food processing industry, such as rancidity resistance.

5.7.3 Proteins

Proteins are the basis of many animal body structures (e.g., muscles, skin, and hair). They also form the enzymes that control chemical reactions throughout the body. Each molecule is composed of amino acids, which are characterized by inclusion of nitrogen and sometimes sulphur (these components are responsible for the distinctive smell of burning protein, such as the keratin in hair). The body requires amino acids to produce new proteins (protein retention) and to replace damaged proteins (maintenance). As there is no protein or amino acid storage provision, amino acids must be present in the diet. Excess amino acids are discarded, typically in the urine. For all animals, some amino acids are essential (an animal cannot produce them internally) and some are non-essential (the animal can produce them from other nitrogen-containing compounds).

Twenty-one proteinogenic amino acids are found in the human body, along with non-proteinogenic amino acids (e.g., gamma-aminobutyric acid). Ten of the proteinogenic amino acids are essential and, therefore, must be included in the diet. A diet that contains adequate amounts of amino acids (especially those that are essential) is particularly important in some situations: during early development and maturation, pregnancy, lactation, or injury (a burn, for instance). A complete protein source contains all the essential amino acids; an incomplete protein source lacks one or more of the essential amino acids.

Sources of dietary protein include meats, tofu and other soy-products, eggs, legumes, and dairy products such as milk and cheese. Excess amino acids from protein can be converted into glucose and used for fuel through a process called gluconeogenesis. The amino acids remaining after such conversion are discarded.

5.7.4 Minerals

Dietary minerals are the chemical elements required by living organisms, other than the four elements carbon, hydrogen, nitrogen, and oxygen that are present in nearly all organic molecules. The term "mineral" is archaic, since the intent is to describe simply the less common elements in the diet. Some are heavier than the four just mentioned, including several metals, which often occur as ions in the body.

Some dietitians recommend that these be supplied from foods in which they occur naturally or at least as complex compounds, or sometimes even from natural inorganic sources (such as calcium carbonate from ground oyster shells). Some minerals are absorbed much more readily in the ionic forms found in such sources. On the other hand, minerals are often artificially added to the diet as supplements; the most famous is likely iodine in iodized salt which prevents goiter.

5.7.5 Vitamins

Vitamins are recognized as essential nutrients, necessary in the diet for good health. Vitamin D is the exception: it can be synthesized in the skin, in the presence of UVB radiation. Certain vitamin-like compounds that are recommended in the diet, such as carnitine, are thought useful for survival and health, but these are not "essential" dietary nutrients because the human body has some capacity to produce them from other compounds. Moreover, thousands of different phytochemicals have recently been discovered in food (particularly in fresh vegetables), which may have desirable properties including antioxidant activity (see below); however, experimental demonstration has been suggestive but inconclusive. Other essential nutrients that are not classified as vitamins include essential amino acids (see above), choline, essential fatty acids (see above), and the minerals discussed in the preceding section.

Vitamin deficiencies may result in disease conditions, including goitre, scurvy, osteoporosis, impaired immune system, disorders of cell metabolism, certain forms of cancer, symptoms of premature aging, and poor psychological health (including eating disorders), among many others. Excess levels of some vitamins are also dangerous to health (notably vitamin A), and for at least one vitamin, B6, toxicity begins at levels not far above the required amount. Deficient or excess levels of minerals can also have serious health consequences.

Table 5.3 Illnesses caused by improper nutrient consumption.

Nutrients	Deficiency	Excess
Macronutrients		
Calories	Starvation, Marasmus	Obesity, diabetes mellitus, Cardiovascular disease
Simple carbohydrates	Ketoacidosis (in diabetics and some other groups)	diabetes mellitus, Obesity, Cardiovascular disease
Complex carbohydrates	Ketoacidosis (in diabetics and some other groups)	Obesity, Cardiovascular disease (high glycemic index foods)
Protein	kwashiorkor	Rabbit starvation, Ketoacidosis (in diabetics)
Saturated fat	Possible essential fatty acid deficiency	Obesity, Cardiovascular Disease
Trans fat	None	Obesity, Cardiovascular Disease
Unsaturated fat	fat-soluble vitamin deficiency, EFA deficiency	Obesity, Cardiovascular disease
Vitamin A	Xerophthalmia and Night Blindness	Hypervitaminosis A (cirrhosis, hair loss)
Vitamin B_1	Beri-Beri	
Vitamin B_2	Skin and Corneal Lesions	
Niacin	Pellagra	dyspepsia, cardiac arrhythmias, birth defects
Vitamin B_{12}	Pernicious Anemia	
Vitamin C	Scurvy	diarrhoea causing dehydration
Vitamin D	Rickets	Hypervitaminosis D (dehydration, vomiting, constipation)
Vitamin E	neurological disease	Hypervitaminosis E (anticoagulant: excessive bleeding)
Vitamin K	Hemorrhage	

Table 5.3 Contd...

Nutrients	Deficiency	Excess
Macronutrients		
Omega 3 Fats	Cardiovascular Disease	Bleeding, Hemorrhages, Hemorrhagic stroke, reduced glycemic control among diabetics
Omega 6 Fats	None	Cardiovascular Disease, Cancer
Cholesterol	None	Cardiovascular Disease[1]
Calcium	Osteoporosis, tetany, carpopedal spasm, laryngospasm, cardiac arrhythmias	Fatigue, depression, confusion, nausea, vomiting, constipation, pancreatitis, increased urination, kidney stones
Magnesium	Hypertension	Weakness, nausea, vomiting, impaired breathing, and hypotension
Potassium	Hypokalemia, cardiac arrhythmias	Hyperkalemia, palpitations
Sodium	hyponatremia	Hypernatremia, hypertension[1]
Iron	Anemia	Cirrhosis, Hepatitis C, heart disease
Iodine	Goiter, hypothyroidism	Iodine Toxicity, Iodism , (goiter, hypothyroidism)[1]

5.8   ROLE OF PHARMACIST IN FAMILY PLANNING

WHO defined family planning as a way of thinking and living that is adopted voluntarily, upon the basis of knowledge, attitudes and responsible decisions by individuals and couples in order to promote the health and welfare of family group and thus contribute effectively to the social development of a country.

Family planning refers to practices that help individual or couples to attain certain objectives as:

(a)   To avoid unwanted birth.

(b)   To regulate suitable intervals between pregnancies.

(c)   To determine number of addition of children in family.

(d)   To control time at which birth occurs in relation to ages of the parents.

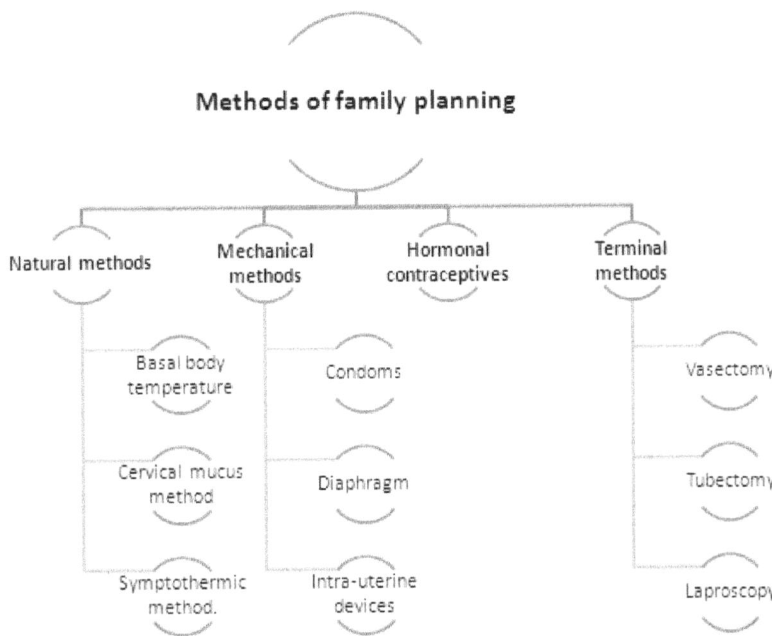

Various methods have been adopted by Government to achieve the desirable results in the program which is the need of the country. Now the ultimate burden lies on to the pharmacists to have adequate participation for success of this program.

(a)   ***Publicity of the program*** and its motives along with methods can be advertised through posters, leaflets and advertisements.

(b)   ***Explanation of techniques*** and solving difficulties of personals interest in acquiring the objectives of the program.

(c)   ***Referral to family planning centers*** about the cases and guide the people to have assistance from health centers for methods and effects.

(d) *Social services* can be made by emphasizing and advising people about the benefits of family planning personally.

(e) *Organizing talks, seminars and documentaries* on family planning as to attract the people to attend and the pharmacist can boost the propaganda of the program.

(f) *Demonstrating the comparative studies* from the nearby society between the family who adopted the program and who has not adopted the program.

PHARMACOECONOMICS AND PHARMACOEPIDEMIOLOGY

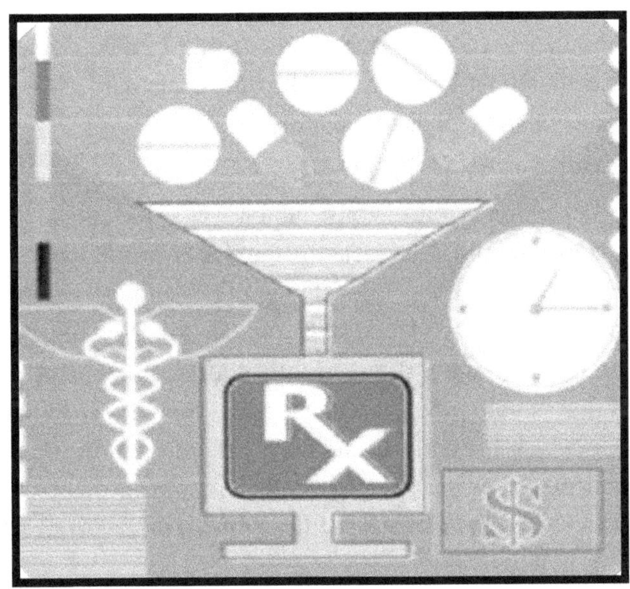

6.1   PHARMACOECONOMICS

Economics is the study of allocation of limited resources or inputs among alternatives uses to satisfy unlimited wants for outputs.

Health economics is the field of study that evaluates the behavior of individuals, firms and markets in health care, and that usually focuses on costs (input) and consequences (outcomes) of health care interventions such as the use of drugs, devices, procedures, services and programs.

Pharmacoeconomics was originally established as a sub-discipline of health economics. Health economics and its branch, pharmacoeconomics, must be considered as means to solve one of the basic questions asked to Health Institutions, namely: how to make a balance between costs for health services and the expected benefits of them. The aim is a maximum health benefit for the community to be delivered considering the existing limited financial resources. The economic evaluations help the health professionals to choose best by the employing various pharmacoeconomic tools.

Pharmacoeconomics is a tool of management which should be applied to strategic and operational decisions about pharmaceutical development, production or consumption. The focus of emphasis in the earliest phase is on informing decisions about product development (essentially go/no go decisions) whilst the emphasis at the later stage shifts to rational prescribing and utilization. The aim throughout is to ensure the most efficient use of limited resources. On the whole pharmacoeconomics should be thought of as an ongoing process which not only bridges the existing gap between R & D and marketing departments of the pharmaceutical companies, but perhaps more importantly, is likely to change the structure of the industry from within.

6.1.1 Introduction

The cost of pharmaceuticals has increased to the double folds in the last five years. Although this growth is predicted to continue in the near future, it is expected to moderate. Those most concerned by rising pharmaceutical costs are, of course, those responsible for paying for and managing these costs. Payers of pharmaceuticals include employers, managed care organizations, and a myriad of health care institutions such as inpatient hospitals etc. Those responsible for managing these costs are the individuals within these institutions, who, through their own expertise and with the help of outside management organizations, such as pharmacy benefit management (PBM) companies, attempt to manage pharmacy costs in the face of limited budgets.

Pharmacoeconomics is a subdivision of health economics and results from that discipline coming of age through consolidation to diversification. Health economics, as a branch of economics is itself relatively young. One can hardly find any systematic reference to it before the mid 1960's and the first reading book on this subject was published in 1973. Pharmacoeconomics is a term used to describe a compilation of methods that evaluate the economic, clinical and humanistic dimensions of pharmaceutical products and services. It is the field of study that evaluates the behavior of individuals, firms and markets relevant to the use of pharmaceutical products, services, programs, and which frequently focuses on the costs (inputs) and consequences (outcomes) of the use. In its most simplistic form, a pharmacoeconomic evaluation compares the economic resources consumed (inputs) to produce the health and economic consequences of products or services (outcomes). This relationship is presented graphically in Fig. 6.1.

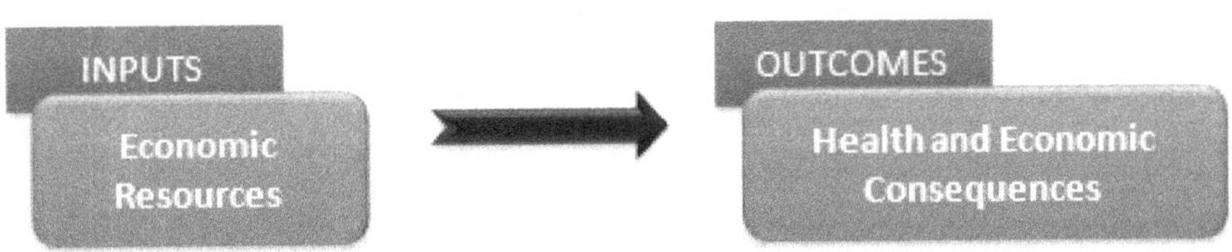

Fig. 6.1 Economic Evaluation of Health Care

Pharmacoeconomics can aid in the decision making in evaluating the affordability and access to the right medication to the right patient at right time, comparing two drugs in the same therapeutic class or drugs with similar mechanism of action and in establishing accountability that the claims by a manufacturer regarding a drug are justified. Some specific scenarios may involve deciding the following:

- Whether a drug should be included in a hospital formulary.

- Which drug would provide net positive benefits to a particular group of patients?

- Which would be the best drug for a pharmaceutical manufacturer to develop and the right price to market it?

- What is the expected quality of life improvement with a certain drug when trading-off its side effects?

The various questions that a reader should ask when appraising a pharmacoeconomic study include:

- What is the perspective of the study?

- What type of study it is?

- Were the competing treatment alternatives described and compared?

- Were the relevant costs and consequences for each alternative properly identified?

- Were the relevant costs and consequences for each alternative properly measured?

- Were the relevant costs and consequences properly valued?

- Were the instruments used to measure patient preferences or quality of life validated?

- What are the assumptions and limitations of the study?

- Were cost and consequences adjusted for different time periods?

- Was a sensitivity analysis performed?

- Are the generalizations appropriate?

6.1.2 Steps for Conducting a Pharmacoeconomic Evaluation

Key components

The main components that must be considered in any pharmacoeconomic evaluation are (Fig. 6.2):

- perspective (health trust, governmental body, insurance company, patients, society in general);

- time horizon;

- cost (direct medical costs, direct nonmedical costs, indirect costs, intangible costs); and

- outcome (years of life saved, years of disease-free survival, cure rate).

Outcome

It is generally considered that there are four principal outcomes of pharmacoeconomic studies:

(i)   Lower cost, better outcome

(ii)   Higher cost, better outcome

(iii)   Lower cost, poorer outcome

(iv)   Higher cost, poorer outcome

It is of course conceivable that a given drug could cost more or less than its competitor while resulting in the same outcome. Clearly, the first outcome is the most favourable for the use of the new treatment. Conversely, the last outcome does not favour the use of the new drug. When the second or third outcome arises, the choice of treatment is up to the prescribing doctor, prescribing policy and the budget available. In such situations, it is also necessary to look at other differences between agents that may sway the decision to prescribe one drug rather than another. These differences may include pharmacokinetic and pharmacodynamic traits, the risk of drug interactions and compliance rates.

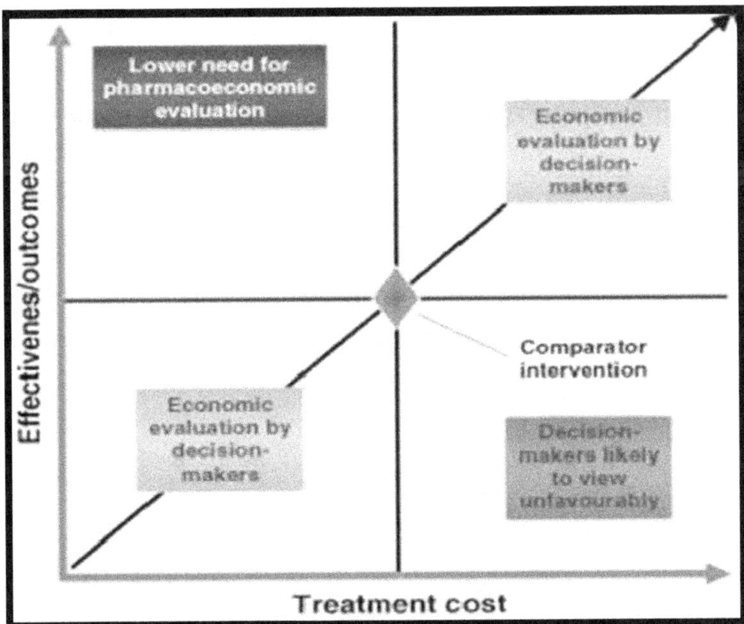

Fig. 6.2 When are pharmacoeconomic analysis needed?

The list of the points that need to be considered when conducting a Pharmacoeconomic evaluation includes (Fig. 6.3):

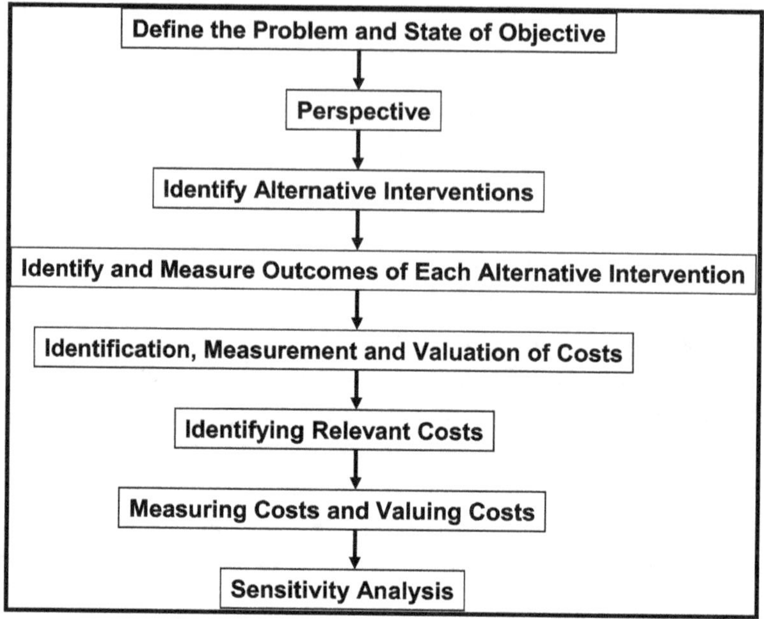

Fig. 6.3 Various steps for conducting a Pharmacoeconomic Evaluation

However, if a Pharmacoeconomic evaluation comprises comparing two or more alternatives and attempts to link costs and effects then these are considered full-economic evaluations. The five major types of full-economic evaluations are:

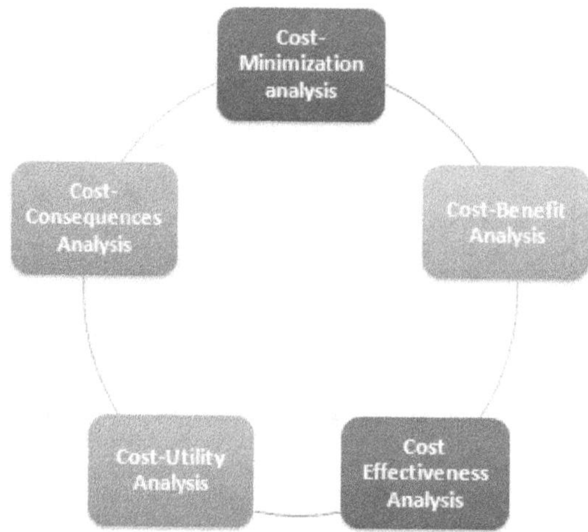

6.1.2.1 Cost-minimization analysis (CMA)

When two or more drugs or alternative programs or interventions have demonstrated equivalent impact in terms of the consequences of an intervention, only the costs of the alternatives need to be compared. Such a cost analysis results in identifying the least costly alternative in terms of monetary value and hence, can be considered as a special case of CEA. Since the primary assumption for cost minimization analysis is that the outcomes of the alternatives are not different, it is imperative that the equivalency of outcomes be established based on valid information such as concurrent trials, published studies in peer reviewed articles or information available form clinical trials.

6.1.2.2 Cost benefit analysis (CBA)

A CBA analysis compares the total costs of each alternative to resultant consequences or benefits of the interventions measured in monetary units. Benefits are measured using contingent valuation also commonly referred to as the willingness to pay method (WTP).

CBA can be used to compare the value alternatives whose outcomes are in different units. The monetary value of the consequences and costs are converted to their net present value by a process called discounting and then compared as net benefit (benefit-costs) or as a ratio (benefit/costs).

6.1.2.3 Cost-effective analysis (CEA)

Cost-effectiveness analysis is a technique used to aid in decision-making between alternatives; when the costs are measured in monetary terms but the consequences are measured in natural unit changes in health. The definition of cost-effectiveness is 'having an additional benefit worth the additional cost'.

6.1.3 Case Studies

Few of the significant case studies highlighting the role of pharmacoeconomics are given below:

6.1.3.1 Formulary decision-making

The use of pharmacoeconomic evaluations for formulary decision-making has become increasingly common. When a new drug is being considered for inclusion on a formulary, the drug is compared with other available alternatives with respect to efficacy & effectiveness, safety and cost. One such study includes with currently available triptans, which offers clear evidence of improved clinical and economic (cost saving) outcomes compared with that of the other abortive migraine therapies, such as ergotamine alkaloids; however, the clinical and economic benefits of triptans are less clear. Such case study introduces a systematic methodology to help formulary decision makers in evaluating the cost-effectiveness of drugs within a category by relying on readily available data.

6.1.3.2 Cost of illness

Peptic ulcer: A 1989 survey on digestive diseases found that ulcers were associated with annual expenditure of US$ 5.65 billion because 40% of patients with ulcers had visited a physician at least five times during the twelve months before the study. Thus, opportunities existed for overall cost savings from better treatment of ulcers.

6.1.3.3 Cost benefit

Influenza vaccination: Evaluation of influenza vaccination among the elderly in New Zealand was quantified in monetary terms the plans' benefits and costs, and their difference or net benefit. Several iterations of this analysis allowed the net benefit of influenza vaccination of the elderly to be considered from a number of different prospective.

6.1.3.4 Cost-effectiveness

ACE-inhibitors in post-myocardial infarction: Comparison of the relative cost-effectiveness of alternative therapies represents this research tool's primary application, as exemplified by a study of angiotensin-converting enzyme (ACE) inhibitors after myocardial infarction. The ratio of cost for each year of life gained varied with the drug cost, indicating strategies for maximizing the use of ACE inhibitors in this high-risk group.

6.1.3.5 Cost utility

Treatment of breast cancer: Women with anthracycline-resistant breast cancer, for example, typically survive with only up to nine months; hence, a therapy that can improve the quality of remaining life can be crucially important. Two treatments for this severe form of breast cancer, namely, docetaxel and paclitaxel were compared using a QALY (Quality Adjusted Life Year) calculated from the patient's preference for health states and treatment outcomes. A slight advantage for docetaxel over paclitaxel, although only about 0.09 QALY per patient, translated into 33 days of perfect meaningful health for patients with only nine months to live.

There is no public health system in the world that has enough resources required for satisfying its full potential. The continuously increasing costs in public health and the limited financial resources for its various implementations demand a judicious allocation of the available resources and their optimal use to achieve effectiveness in health services. Pharmacoeconomics, like a multi-discipline action field, unites the efforts of clinical pharmacologists, pharmacists, health economists, epidemiologists and others in search of a balance between the costs for health services and their results. It compares the costs and consequences (outcomes) of drug therapies and medical interventions and also guides choices among alternative medications, treatment regimens and services based on a combination of costs and outcomes.

6.2 PHARMACOEPIDEMIOLOGY

It is the application of epidemiological reasoning, methods and knowledge to study the beneficial (therapeutic) and adverse effects of a drug in a set of human population. The results of these interventions may be positive or negative.

6.2.1 Aims and Applications of Pharmacoepidemiology

- *Identification of adverse drug reactions* using various methods of pharmacoepidemiology both pre-marketing and post-marketing.

- *Identification of drug-risk benefit*: **R**isk includes the prediction of both attributable risk and relative risk associated with the drugs.

- *Qunatification of outcomes*: It is very important in order to predict the major risk and benefits involved in dispensing and administration of drugs.

- *Pharmacoviligance* is the branch of pharmacoepidemiology which is defined as the post approval scientific and data gathering activities related to the detection, assessment, understanding and prevention of adverse events or other product related problems.

Consequences of drug use include:

- *Negative outcomes* which refers to adverse drug events. This involves the relationship between drug ingestion and a subsequent negative outcome.

- ***Positive outcome*** refers to efficacy (clinical effects of drugs when used under ideal conditions like ideal patient monitoring, complete control of interfering factors etc.) or effectiveness (drug use under normal condition of day to day life) of the drugs.

6.2.2 Levels of Pharmacoepidemological Studies

There are three levels of pharmacoepidemological studies:

- Micro-level

- Macro level and

- Meso level

6.2.2.1 Micro level

It reflects the measurement at the level of individual patients, prescribers or pharmacists. In fact this level is single-subject based interpretation.

6.2.2.2 Macro level

It refers to usual level which refers to that of population and deals with processes as pattern of drug use in the population, overall net benefit of drug use in the society, expenditure on drugs at national and international level and drug policy.

6.2.2.3 Meso level

It refers to that group of people, who are clustered together by a common factor, such as age (e.g. geriatric people), geography, drug use, disease, services etc. In fact this level if specific-subject class base interpretation.

So pharmacoepidemology is concerned with identifying patterns of drug use, consequences and factors that may help to explain and understand these phenomenons.

6.2.3 Types of Studies

Fundamental studies on the basis of method in which subjects are arranged to treatments

- ***Experimental studies*****:** Investigator assigns treatment to subject either randomly or in the form of analytical or descriptive studies.

- ***Non-experimental studies*****:** No assignments of treatment to subject by investigator. In this studies enroll patients receiving care, including medications from conventional settings.

Table 6.1 Experimental Studies

Study type	Description	Number of patients (per treatment group)	Example
Randomized clinical trials	Study patients with specific disease	50 to 5000	Efficacy of altiplase and retiplase in preventing death after myocardial infarction
Field trials	Study subject to prevent disease	>5000	Vaccination to prevent polio
Community intervention trials	Study communities to prevent diseases	>5000	Fluorination of water to prevent dental caries

Table 6.2 Non Experimental Studies

Prospective cohort	Observe group of patients treated with the same drug	**>5000**	Nurses study health study cohort
Retrospective cohort	Extract data from an existing respository to look at outcomes of exposed groups	>5000	Risk of renal insufficiency from NSAIDs
Case control	Determine association between drug and rare event	20 to 1000	Risk of alzheimer's disease and vitamin use
Case series	Reveal common experiences of a number of patients following drug exposure	3 to 30	Valvular heart disease associated with fen fluramine phentirmine (Fen-Phen)
Case report	Experience of single patient following drug exposure	1	Toxic epidermal necrolysis from phenytoin
Trend analysis	Determine past case history of patient	1	
Cross sectional	Determine prevelance of drug use in patient population at a time	50 to 1 million	Profile of calcium channel antagonists in a managed-care organization.

6.2.4 Advantages and Disadvantages of Pharmacoepidemiological Studies

6.2.4.1 Randomized control trials

(a) Advantages

- It is used to compare the efficacy of two or more drugs.
- It also determines whether drugs differ in their propensity to cause adverse drug reaction.

(b) Disadvantages

- *Prohibitively expensive*: The costs normally is in million, so it is rarely conducted.
- *Unethical*: These are unethical for studies of ADR as the effects of drugs are to be studied on patients by deliberately exposures.
- Large number of subjects required to carry out the study.
- Time consuming.

6.2.4.2 Cohort studies and prospective studies

Cohort studies involve cohort which are the group of patients having common drug exposure of interest while prospective studies looks forward in time.

(a) Advantages

- The event of interest is specifically defined and monitored.
- Explanation of potential compounding factors and variables is carried out and they are also measured.

(b) Disadvantages

- Expensive

6.2.4.3 Retrospective cohort

These studies look back on existing data.

(a) Advantages

- Cheaper
- It also leads to pretime studies.

(b) Disadvantages

Involvement of extensive biasing: A number of biasing is involved in this study which is difficult to remove.

6.2.4.4 Case control study

Diametric opposite of cohort studies. Cases are group of patients with common disease while control refers to people who are representatives of underlying population contributing the cases.

(a) Advantages

- Access to rare outcome.

- Less expensive.

- Require less number of subjects. Access to multiple exposures on single outcome.

(b) Disadvantages: Rare outcome is most desirable aspect but it creates problem for investigator to find the rare outcomes.

Investigator begins by assembling group of patients having outcome of interest and then match on important variables e.g. Age, sex or disease severity with similar group of individuals who did not have that outcome. Such may occur with orphan drugs.

6.2.4.5 Case reports

Best for detecting rare or unusual reactions that occur during initial or prolonged drug use and are major source for generating hypothesis about adverse drug reactions e.g. Action of minoxidil as a hair growth stimulant by zappacosta.

(a) Advantages

- Vital for rare outcomes because no other studies can contribute so much to this filed.

- Focusing on initial and prolonged drug use is the main feature of this study that imports a unique character to this study.

(b) Disadvantages

- Subject to bias and errors as they develop reporter bias and erroneous reporting.

- *Inpredictable to increase in reactions*: Although it is involving ADRs and other drug problems but it cannot predict the enhancement in reactions that occur remotely in time from the actual drug use.

- No relation between prescribing patterns and reporting rates is one of the main limitations of this study.

6.2.4.6 Case series

Case series is a set of sequential case reports identified either by exposure or outcome e.g. Adverse drug events like weight gain, sedation and akathisia in childern was confirmed by report of Krishnamurthi and King on use of olanzapine.

(a) Advantages

- Knowledge enrichment regarding drug use and their consequences as it involves a number of patients for study.

- Open trial of drug is very satisfactory for investigator.

(b) Disadvantages

Lack of formal trial protocol.

6.2.4.7 Trend analysis

Trend analysis involve plotting of data over time with the help of which the past case history of patient can be detected e.g. Iif we plot use of antibiotics over time and number of resistant strains of bacteria developed over the same time frame. The shift in trend line suggests the change in relationship.

(a) Advantages

- Data dynamics visualization is the main feature of this study. This leads to a clear idea to reader regarding the pattern.

- Trend Linkage- such trend analysis suggests that events may be linked however the observer must beware.

6.2.4.8 Database studies

An ideal database have all requisite data for conducting pharmacoepidemological research including information on patient, diagnosis, drug and outcomes.

(a) Advantages

- *Versatility*: Researchers can conduct any type of observational study under this database.

- *Accurate estimation of ADR incidences*: Because it can contain data from literally millions of patients.

- Estimation of rate of drug effectiveness or comparative patient outcomes such as death or cost of care.

(b) Disadvantages

- Miscoded data is the limitation of data base weather it is paper based.

- Lack of important information because they were developed for purposes other than pharmacoepidemologic research. As data base insurance have information other than diagnosis or patient characteristics.

6.2.5 Measuring Drug Use: Units of Use

Measuring the drug use in terms of cost effectiveness and drug is usually expressed as proportion where numerator is expresses in utilization and denominator as a variety of units.

6.2.5.1 Monetary unit

Everything can be easily translated into monetary terms (like dollars, pounds, rupees) and in turn can be converted into other units.

(a) Advantages

- Flexible system as every term can be translated into this unit and vice-versa.

- ***Discounted over time***: They can be easily discounted over time regularly.

(b) Disadvantages

- No measure of actual drug use, one cannot determine as how many people are using how much of drug.

- Unprediction of monetary value of drug scale means in terms of quantity of drug consumed.

6.2.5.2 In prescription terms

It is the straight forward and simple unit to express and understand. It describes that what drug to be dispensed how many times. This is a simple method as it does not involve any special criteria for expression.

- **Disadvantages:**

  Variation in dispensing factor prediction as it cannot explain strength of drug, price of drug, price fluctuations over time and geography.

  Variation in drug utilization techniques: Every prescriber has his own considerations for a particular drug which directly influences the prescription strategy.

6.2.5.3 Number of units of drugs

These are the units of drugs refers to number of tablets, capsules etc. dispensed and consumed.

- **Advantages**

  Determination of quantity individual drug dispensed, as it helps to predict the quantity of tablets, capsules etc. at sale.

  *Prediction of most compliant ones***:** The dosage form at highest sale is the most compliant to patients.

6.2.5.4 Defined daily dose (DDD)

It is a technical unit of measurement developed by WHO in 1993. It is based on average daily dose of drug when used in adults for its major indications. Utilization is most often reported in countries as DDD per 1000 inhabitants of that country and in hospitals as DDD per 100 bed days.

This approach was first used by Srishyla et al. in 1994 for a hospital in Bangalore.

(a) **Advanatges**

- It is a uniform concept that can be applied to a number of drugs.
- Compare in-country drug utilization and also interregional utilization and helps to have across on drug therapy fluctuation according to geography.

(b) **Disadvantages**

- Non applicable to pediatrics drugs.
- Lack of versatalities as it cannot be applicable to all drugs.

6.2.5.5 Outcome measures of drug

- **Prevalence** is the proportion of people affected by or exposed to a drug at a given time.
- *Statistics involved*: Cross sectional statistics which is determined by means of survey.
- *Range of value*: Prevalence can vary between 0 and 1 and is expressed as cases per 1000 exposures or per 1000 inhabitants.
- *Prevalence point* is the prevalence at any given time.
- *Annual prevalence* is the prevalence for a year example in a city total population is around 2000 and people effected = 4000 so the prevalence ratio = 4000/200000 = **0.02**.

- *Cumulative incidence*is referred to simply as 'incidence'. These are the number of new cases of disease or outcome that occur in a population in a specific defined time period divided by total number of people in that population. It is longitudinal measure which is time dependent and is normally measured with an inception cohort study.

  Cumulative incidence is expressed either as a percentage or proportion per unit time (e.g. Cases per 1000 population per year).

  Relation between prevalence and cumulative incidence:

  *** Prevalence = Incidence × Average duration of disease***

- **Incidence rate or Incidence density**

  It is the number of new cases that appears over the amount of person-time at risk and is most commonly expressed as cases per person-year exposure. For denomination, the time each person was at risk (i.e. taking the drug) is : Σ (person X time exposed) e.g. 5000 people continue to take a NSAIDs for 7 years, 4000 people continue to take it for 4 years, out of total 1000 of them developed gastrointestinal bleeding denominator = 5000 X 7 + 4000 X 4 = 35000 + 16000 = 51000

  $$Ratio = 1000/51,000$$

6.2.5.6 Risk

It is the probability of developing an outcome when exposed to a drug. It is independent of seriousness, severity or harm. Each outcome has its own risk which depends on a number of factors like age, sex, physiological condition of patient, co-morbidities etc. For example, Nicotine gum has a risk for providing hiccups but outcome are not harmful.

They are of two types

(i) *Attributable risk:* It is the statistic that is simple to calculate, understand and expressed clinically as rate difference. It quantifies how much higher one rate is than that of its comparator. For example, If one drug is 80% successful and another is 65% successful, the rate difference is 15%.

(ii) *Relative Risk or Risk ratio:* It is the ratio of the rate of outcomes in a non-exposed comparison group. Rate ratio = Rate $_{exposed}$/ Rate $_{non-exposed}$ example if 40 out of 1000 people receiving a drug develop a rash, as compared with 20 out of 1000 who did not take the drug.

$$Relative\ Risk = 40/1000 \div 20/1000 = 2$$

It means people taking the drug develop the rashes twice as often as do people who do not take the drug.

	Outcome	*No outcome*	*Total*
Persons exposed	A	B	C_1
Persons non-exposed	C	D	C_0
Total	C_1	C_0	N

Presentation of results from pharmacoepidemological studies

Relative risk: $A/\{(A+B) \div (C/C+D)\}$

Table 6.3 Types of measurements in pharmacoepidemological studies

Measure	*Definition*	*Comments*
Prevalence	Frequency of cases at a given time or period	Often confused with incidence reported as percentage
Point prevalence	Frequency of cases at an instant	Used in cross-sectional studies
Period prevalence	Frequency of cases within a period as one year	Confused with point prevalence
Incidence	Frequency of new cases in a population over a period	Mostly reported as rate as 10/10,000 persons/year
Relative risk ratio	Incidence is the exposed group to the incidence in unexposed group	Addresses the number of times greater risk in exposed than in unexposed; a relative risk of one means risk is equal with or without exposure
Odds ratio	It is the probability of an outcome happening divided by the probability of event not happening. An odd ratio is the odds of events in those exposed divided by odds in unexposed	Provides an estimate of relative risk for rate outcome; an odds ratio of one means that there is no association between exposure and outcome
Attributable risk	Incidence in exposed group – incidence in unexposed group	Addresses the incidence of a disease attributed to an exposure

6.2.6　Evidence Based Management (EBM) and its Co-relation with Pharmacoepidemology

On the basis of epidemiological studies choice of drug or medication can be made which are safe and having better and good therapeutic action or effect. According to Sackett et al., EBM can be defined as the integration of best result from evidence with clinical expertise and patient values. EBM is the study which is carried out to bring down maximum safety, effectiveness both in terms of therapeutic activity and cost effectiveness.

RATIONAL DRUG THERAPY

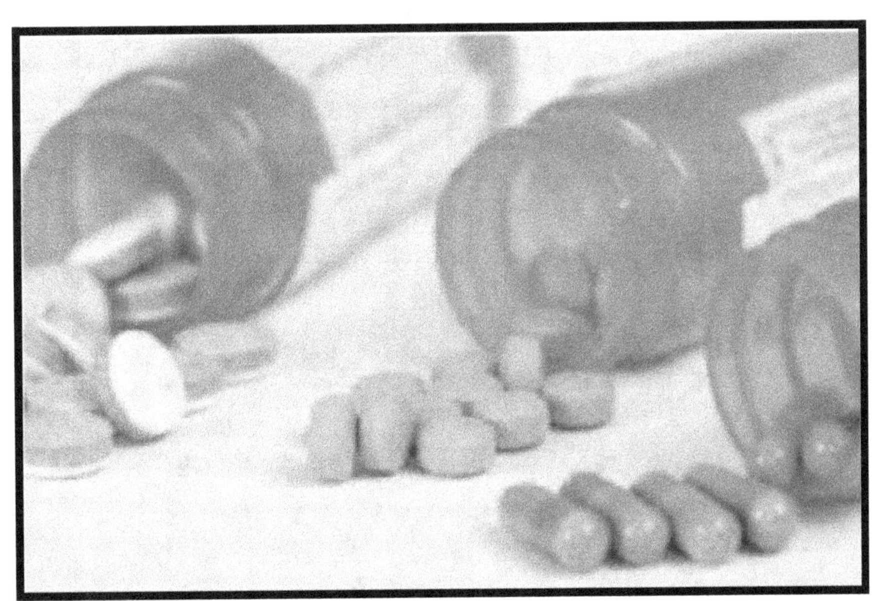

7.1 RATIONAL DRUG THERAPY (RDT)

WHO committee experts discussed various aspects of health care and possibilities to improve them by focusing on various factors such as efficacy, cost, safety and effectiveness of extensive drugs use in most of the countries. This effort lead to development of a list of drugs which were of proven safety, efficacy and effectiveness and possessed well understood therapeutic properties called *essential drugs* and the list is called as *essential drug list*.

WHO definition of essential drugs: "Essential medicines are those that satisfy the priority health care needs of population". They are selected with due regard to public, health relevance, evidence on efficacy, safety and comparative cost effectiveness. Essential medicines are the drugs that have the best balance of quality, safety, efficacy and cost for a given ailment and are needed at most to cure majority of ailment in a population.

7.1.1 Objectives of Rational Drug Therapy

1. To maximize effectiveness and safety of medications.

2. To identify patients requiring proper counseling.

3. To minimize the risk of medication errors.

4. To maintain equilibrium among explanatory factors for rational drug therapy.

5. To provide indiscriminate medications to all.

6. To make a check on economy related to health care.

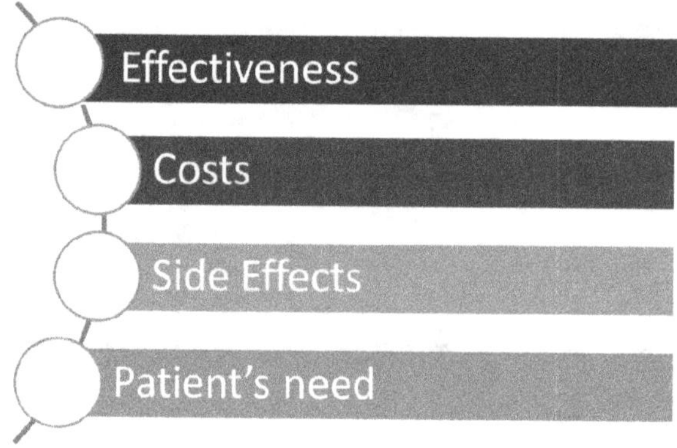

Fig. 7.1 Inter-relation of various Objectives of Rational Drug Therapy.

7.1.2 Factors Stimulating the Concept of Essential Drugs

    (a) Limited access to medicines essential to meet the health needs of majority of population.

    (b) Limited public functioning for pharmaceuticals and health.

In 1977: 1st model was published and has since been updated every two years. The list comprises of 220 medicines.

In 1999: WHO expert committee of essential medicines reviewed current procedures for updating the model list.

In 2002: 11th model list of essential medicines was revised by expert committee using new procedures.

The 12th model list of essential medicines contains 325 medicines for the treatment of various infectious and chronic diseases. The updated model list has two lists:

Core list indicating minimum drug needs for a basic health care system and ***Compliment list*** includes mainly essential medicines for priority diseases which may be cost effective but not necessarily affordable.

The latest model list reflects a model product, developed through a model process and both models can be used for advocacy purposes.

Normally a drug treatment process is regarded under two perspectives:

    (i) *Macro-perspective* which include an analysis of different systems and structural components in place to ensure use of drugs.

    (ii) *Micro-perspective* includes patient level and interaction between the patient and the practitioner.

7.1.3 Principles of Essential Drug Concept

7.1.3.1 Maximum treatment with minimum medicines

Common health problems of majority of population can be treated with small and carefully selected medicines.

7.1.3.2 Adequate drug utilization

Health professionals routinely used less than 200 medicines. Training and clinical experiences should focus on proper use of these selected medicines.

7.1.3.3 Economic and efficient carrying out activities

Procurement, distribution and other supply activities can be carried out most economically and efficiently for a limited number of drug problems.

7.1.3.4 Proper information to patients

Patients can be better informed about the effective use of medicines by the health professionals.

7.1.4 Role of Pharmacist in Rational Drug Therapy (RDT)

7.1.4.1 Counseling of patients and physician

The counseling about the new drugs variation in drug policy, availability of drugs etc. should be provided timely to the patient and the physician. Patient should be counseled about proper drug use.

7.1.4.2 Stating adverse effects of drugs

Adverse drug reactions should be reported to proper monitoring centers in hospitals, region or country. Prescribers should be informed about ADRs by the pharmacists.

7.1.4.3 Drug procurement

The selection and range of drugs should be based on essential drug concept in accordance to the needs and situation. Procurement of most cost effective drugs in right quantities and there should be selection of reliable suppliers of high quality products. Delivery should be timely and lowest possible total cost should be achieved.

7.1.4.4 List preparation

Pharmacist as being a drug representative in public can state about the physico-social requirements of the prevailing population and can contribute to prepare the most cost effective list.

7.1.4.5 Inventory control

Monitoring of the drug stocks and minimizing 'out of stock' situations should be carried out. Drug formulary should be properly used. Essential drugs should be maintained in over stock.

7.1.4.6 Pharmaceutical care

An evidenced based approach, weighing the pros and cons of treatment, monitoring of treatment outcomes, suggestions to modify treatment plan are the responsibilities of pharmacist. Aim of the care is to optimize the patients health related quality of life and achieve cost effective clinical outcomes.

7.1.4.7 Promotion of RDU

It can be done by arranging discussions on new drugs and changing strategies/ treatment need through questionnaire techniques, video clipping techniques, seminars etc. by the pharmacist.

7.2   IMPACT OF ESSENTIAL DRUGS

Cost effective tools for fighting ill-health are available in the form of Essential drugs and the impact of essential drugs include:

(i)   **Health impact**

Essential drug treatments are available for most prevailing communicable diseases like malaria, T.B., AIDS, acute respiratory infections and diarrhoeal diseases. Essential lives saving medicines are available for non-communicable diseases like ischemic heart disease and cerebrovascular diseases. The availability of essential medications has been found to attract patients to health facilities, unless they can also benefit from preventive services.

(ii)   **Economic impact**

In high income countries the cost of medicines is not directly borne by the patient as $2/3^{rd}$ of medicines are pre-paid through Government revenues and social-health insurance program. In middle income countries, public spending on medicines represents the largest health expenditure while in the low income countries, 50-90% of the medicines are paid out of pocket at the time of illness and represents largest non-budgeted household expenditure. By focusing on pharmaceutical expenditure on essential medicines, the cost effectiveness of Government and personal outlay drug expenditure can be improved and health impact strengthened.

7.2.1 Essential Drug indicators

These are the indicators described by World Health Organization (WHO) in 1993 to serve as tools to select the essential drugs and as measures to monitor the treatment practices, to completely prescribing behavior in different areas or facilities or to access the impact of an intervention designed to improve drug use.

7.2.1.1 Prescribing indicators

  (a) Average number of drugs per prescription.

  (b) Percentage of drugs prescribed by generic name.

  (c) Percentage of encounters with an antibiotic prescribed.

  (d) Percentage of encounters with an injection prescribed.

  (e) Percentage of drugs prescribed from an essential drug list or formulary.

7.2.1.2 Patient care indicators

  (a) Average consultation time.

  (b) Average dispensing time.

  (c) Percentage of drugs actually dispensed.

  (d) Percentage of drugs adequately labeled.

  (e) Patient knowledge of current dosage.

7.2.1.3 Facility indicators

  (a) Availability of copy of essential drug list or formulary.

  (b) Availability of key drugs.

7.2.1.4 Complimentary indicators

  (a) Percentage of patients treated without drugs.

  (b) Average drug cost per encounter.

  (c) Percentage of drug cost spent on antibiotics.

  (d) Percentage of drug cost spent on injections.

(e) Prescription in accordance with treatment guidelines.

(f) Percentage of patients satisfied with the care they received.

(g) Percentage of health facilities with access to impartial information.

7.2.2 Selection of Essential Drugs

The various factors influencing the selection of essential drugs include-

7.2.2.1 Pattern of disease

For communicable disease specific antibiotics, vaccines are to be in focus but for non-communicable diseases life-saving medicines are to be considered.

7.2.2.2 Cost factor

For developing countries drug should be available at most reliable or low cost as compared to those in developed countries.

7.2.2.3 Storage conditions

At places such as high humid, the drugs with hygroscopic nature prove to be a problem for storage. So drugs are to be chosen according to environmental conditions prevailing.

7.2.2.4 Treatment facilities

In backward areas with no proper facilities available, drugs with most efficacy and safety should be recommended.

7.2.2.5 Patient compliance

Drugs should be properly selected according to the need of the patients and ease of administration.

7.2.3 Model List of Essential Drugs

Essential drugs are the list of those medicines which have proved to be the most efficient and cost effective. In a given context these selected medicines are the ones most needed for national health services and be available at all the times in adequate amount and in proper dosage forms.

Essential medicines concept underpinned the fact that a limited range of systematically selected essential medicines stimulate better quality of health care provisions, improves drug management, prescribing, dispensing with low cost.

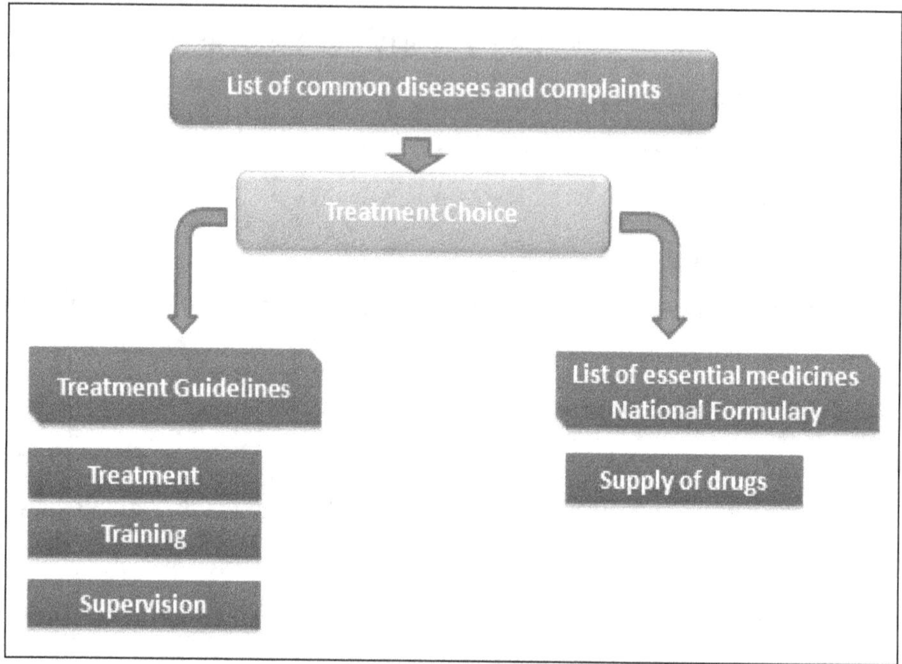

Fig. 7.2 Relationship between treatment guidelines and list of essential medicines.

7.2.4 Evaluation of Irrational Use of Drugs

Impact of irrational use of drugs can be evaluated as,

7.2.4.1 Diminished quality of drug therapy

Irrational drugs causes diminished quality of life to patients and improper combinations, dosage regimen and doses causes decreased quality of drug therapy.

7.2.4.2 Psychological impact

It leads to a drug phobia like attitude towards drug therapy.

7.2.4.3 Wastage of resources

Resources also get wasted as the patient has to spend more on medication therapy for same medication if it was rational.

7.2.4.4 Increased risk of unwanted effects

Unwanted effects like adverse drug reactions (ADRs), emergency drug resistance etc. are the major ones.

7.2.5 Irrational Prescribing Practice

Irrational prescribing practice involves:

7.2.5.1 Prescribing drugs with no value

Prescribing drugs with no value is common among the psychologically ill patients but not adequate for all the patients as it betrays the basic health needs of the patient.

7.2.5.2 Prescription for self-limiting conditions

Prescription for self-limiting conditions like cough, cold etc. can pose a monetary profit to the prescriber but on part of the patient, it bring various long term complications.

7.2.5.3 Over doing and under dosing

Over doing and under dosing is one of the major medication errors which either contributes to ADRs or not produce any effect. This mainly occurs due to wrong calculations and predications.

7.2.5.4 Preference to costly drugs

Even if the oral formulations are available, some prescribers prefer injectables which are quite expensive and do not meet the patient compliance.

7.2.5.5 Improper dosage regimen and monitoring of the medication chart

Improper dosage regimen and monitoring of the medication chart can bring out certain problems to the patients like ADRs etc.

7.2.6 Activities Involved in Promotion of Rational Drug Use

7.2.6.1 Adoption of essential drug concept

Adoption of essential drug concept as it helps in selecting the best therapy among the available better once after concerning and comparing all the vital factors such as efficacy, safety, effectiveness and cost.

7.2.6.2 Counseling of health professionals in RDT

Counseling of health professionals in RDT is essential to maintain updated knowledge and concepts regarding the available therapy and medicines to be delivered.

7.2.6.3 Development of evidence-based clinical guidelines

Development of evidence-based clinical guidelines provides the best access to the prevailing diseases and predicting out its best therapy.

7.2.6.4 Consumer education

Consumer education plays a crucial role in the promotion of rational drug use.

BIBLIOGRAPHY

1. Ansel H.C., *Introduction to Pharmaceutical Dosage Forms*, Lea and Febiger, Philadelphia.

2. Gennaro A.R., *Remington's Pharmaceutical Sciences*, 20th Edition, 2000, Mac Publishing Co., Easton, Philadelphia, PA.

3. Lachman L., Lieberman H.A., Kaing J.L., *The Theory and Practice of Industrial Pharmacy*, Lea and Febiger, Philadelphia.

4. Banker G.S. and Chalmers R.K., *Pharmaceutics and Pharmacy Practice*, Lippincott.

5. D. M. Brahamankar and Sunil B. Jaiswal; Biopharmaceutics and Pharmacokinetics: A Treatise, 1st Edition, Vallabh Prakashan, Delhi.

6. Leon Shargelet.al. *Pharmacy Review*, A Wiley Medical Publication, John Wiley and Sons, Singapore.

7. Pashos C.L., Klein E.G. and Wanke L.A., 1998, ISPOR Lexicon, 1st Edition, *International Society for Pharmacoeconomics and Outcomes research*, Princeton, NJ.

8. C.V.S. Subramanyam, *Pharmaceutical Production and Management*, VallabhPrakashan, New Delhi.

9.   G Parthasarthi, Karin Nyfort-Hansen and Milap C Nahata, *Cliniacl Pharmacy Paractice: Essential Concepts and Skills*, Orient Longman private Limited, Chennai, 2004.

10. Nakahiro R.K., Ho S.S.and Okamoto M, Concepts of Pharmacoeconomics. In.,MirtaMillares (Ed.) *Applied Drug Information: Strategies for information management.* Applied Therapeutics, Inc. Vancouver, Canada, 1998.

11. Kamal Dua, U.V.Singh Sara, Vijay Kumar Sharma, AbhinavAgrawal, M.V.Ramana, "OTC Medications: Relevance and Significance for Consumers", *The Indian Pharmacist*, Vol.6 (55): 47-49, 2007 (Annual Issue).

12. Kamal Dua, Vijay Kumar Sharma, U.V.Singh Sara, AbhinavAgrawal, M.V.Ramana, J.C. Dua, "Pediatric OTC Medications: Vital Consideration", *The Indian Pharmacist,* Feb 2007, Vol.6, No.56: 23-27.

13. Kamal Dua, Vijay Kumar Sharma, U.V.Singh Sara, M.V. Ramana, "Pharmacist: An Indispensable Safety Reservoir for OTC Medications", *The Indian Pharmacist*, Vol.6, No.59: 28-30, 2007.

14. Roger Walker and Clive Edwards, *Clinical Pharmacy and Therapeutics*, 3rd Edition, Churchill Livingstone, New York.

15. S.GeorgeCarruthers, Brian B.Hoffman, Kenneth L. Melmon and David W Nierenberg, *Clinical Pharmacology: Melmon and Morrellis*, 4th Edition, Mc-Graw Hill, New York.

16. N.K. Jain, *Health Education & Community Pharmacy*, CBS Publishers and Distributors, New Delhi.

17. Stoller E.P., Prescribed and over-the-counter medicine used by the ambulatory elderly, *Med. Care*, 26, 1988, 1149-57.

18. N.K. Jain, Text Book of *Forensic Pharmacy* (6th Ed.) VallabhPrakashan Delhi.

19. A.K. Gupta, *Handbook of Health Education and Community Pharmacy*, CBS Publishers and Distributors, New Delhi.

20. Derck G Walker, Andrew G. Renwick and Keith Hillier, *Medical Pharmacology and Therapeutics*, Ist Edition, Saunders, New York.

21. Janie Sheridan, *Drug Misuse and Community Pharmacy*, CRC Press, USA.

22. Mei-Jen Ho, Vijay N. Joish and Joseph E. Biskupiak, P&T, The Role of Pharmacoeconomics in Formulary Management: Triptan Case Study for Migraine, P&T, January 2005. Vol. 30 No. 1, 36-46.

23. Sonnenberg A., J.E. Everhart, Health Impact of Peptic Ulcers in the United States, American Journal of Gastroenterology, 92 (4), 1997, 614-620.

24. Scott W.G. and Scott H.M., Economic Evaluation of Vaccination against Influenza in New Zealand, Pharmacoeconomics, 1996, 9 (1), 51-60.

25. McMurray J.J., McGuire A., A.P. Davie and H. Hughes, Cost-Effectiveness of Different ACE Inhibitor Treatment Scenarios Post-Myocardial Infarction, European Heart Journal, 18 (9), 1997, 1411-1415.

26. G.C. Yee, Cost-Utility Analysis of Taxane Therapy, American Journal of Health Systems and Pharmacy, 54, 24 Suppl 2, 1997, S11-S15.

27. http://en.wikipedia.org/woki/Communication

28. http://askdrwiki.com/mediawiki/index.php?title=Body_plethysmography

29. http://en.wikipedia.org/wiki/Nutrition